Respiratory Infections and Tumours

Roger White, MA, MD, MRCP

Consultant Physician
Frenchay Hospital, Bristol

SPRINGER-SCIENCE+BUSINESS MEDIA, B.V.

ISBN 978-94-009-8089-1   ISBN 978-94-009-8087-7 (eBook)
DOI 10.1007/978-94-009-8087-7

Fakenham Press Limited, Fakenham, Norfolk

Contents

INFECTIONS

1. Introduction

There is a wide variation in the clinical syndromes and in the severity of respiratory tract infections. This diversity is only partly accounted for by the large number of infecting agents, because a particular microorganism can itself result in different illnesses. The age, fitness and state of immunity of the patient is of great relevance, and the clinical features of a particular infection vary accordingly. In terms of incidence of infection the acute virus infections are far in the lead.

Respiratory infections can be broadly classified into acute and chronic. The acute infections are generally due to bacteria, viruses, rickettsiae and mycoplasma. Chronic infection is either bacterial, mycobacterial, fungal or parasitic in origin.

Protection Against Infection

There are three methods by which man can protect himself against infections of the respiratory tract—mechanical barriers, phagocytic cells and the immune response.

Mechanical Barriers

The cough reflex protects the lung against inhaled irritant substances and larger particles. Smaller particles will be trapped by the layer of mucus which covers the respiratory tract. The ciliated epithelium maintains a constant upward flow of the mucus and via this mucociliary escalator expels particles from the respiratory tract.

Infection can occur when these mechanical barriers are altered, and the defect in the mucociliary lining accounts for the increased susceptibility to infection in chronic bronchitis and bronchiectasis.

Phagocytic Cells

There are two types of phagocyte: polymorphonuclear leucocytes and alveolar macrophages. Invading microorganisms cause an inflammatory response which includes the rapid arrival of polymorphs whose function is to phagocytose the organisms. Macrophages are present in much smaller numbers than polymorphs and their function is to clear the cell debris as well as microorganisms. Many microorganisms are able to resist phagocytosis by the production of toxins which kill the cells, as in staphylococcal infection, or alternatively by having a protective coating, such as the capsule of pneumococcus.

The Immune Response

There are two components of the immune response:

1. The humoral response mediated by circulating antibody formed by 'B' (bone marrow) lymphocytes.

2. The cell-mediated response which is expressed by the 'T' (thymus-dependent) lymphocytes.

The Humoral Response

IgA antibody. This is the local protective antibody of the respiratory epithelium. It acquires the 'secretory piece', which is a peptide chain, when it is secreted through the epithelium. The mechanism of action of the antimicrobial antibody of IgA is not completely understood, but it may inhibit the penetration of organisms through the layer of mucus over the respiratory epithelium.

IgM and IgG antibody. The classical response to non-replicating antigens is an initial short-lived increase in IgM, followed by a latent period of a few days and then a larger and more prolonged IgG response.

Most infections are due to replicating antigens and so the antigen stimulus is more prolonged and the primary and secondary immune responses become less distinguishable. The role of the humoral antibodies varies according to the infection, but in outline they have the following properties:

1. They can coat bacteria and make them more susceptible to phagocytosis (opsonization).

2. They can combine with organisms and impair their ability to attach to mucosal cells, as in influenza.

As a result of the combination of antibody with antigen, complement is fixed and this fixing of complement to the organisms has an opsonizing effect and therefore promotes phagocytosis. However, lysis of the organisms can be a direct result of attachment of complement to antibody-coated cells.

Cell-mediated Immunity

Cell-mediated immunity is important in combating organisms, including mycobacteria and viruses, which can live and divide within cells, and are therefore protected against humoral antibodies. This explains the susceptibility of patients with deficient cell-mediated immunity to tuberculosis and serious virus infection whereas, unlike patients with immunoglobulin deficiencies (e.g. chronic lymphatic leukaemia), they can usually withstand bacterial invasion.

T cells can lyse infected cells and can release lymphokines which attract and concentrate macrophages at the site of infection. Interferon is produced when T cells react with antigen, but its role is not clear.

2. Acute Respiratory Infections

The clinical syndromes may be classified according to the part of
the respiratory tract involved:

Upper and middle respiratory tract—
  Common cold (coryza)
  Acute sore throat (pharyngitis and tonsillitis)
  Acute epiglottitis
  Acute laryngitis
  Acute tracheobronchitis
  Influenza
  Whooping cough

Lower respiratory tract—
  Acute bronchiolitis
  Pneumonia

Most infections of the upper respiratory tract are due to viruses,
except acute epiglottitis which is usually caused by *Haemophilus
influenzae.* While some viruses regularly cause characteristic illnesses, there is no set of symptoms which is specific to a particular
virus. These virus infections are very common and are very con-
tagious. Epidemics of varying magnitude are likely to occur, and
are particularly frequent in winter months. Most of the infections are relatively mild, cause discomfort for a few days and pass
without sequelae but they can sometimes predispose to more
serious infection, especially in the infirm and those with pre-
existing lung disease.

Common Cold (Coryza)

A virus can be found in about 50 per cent of cases of common cold; this is usually a rhinovirus or coronavirus, although similar symptoms can result from parainfluenza and respiratory syncytial virus. The onset is often abrupt, and is sometimes preceded by an irritant sensation in the throat. The nasal obstruction, runny nose, sore throat and conjunctivitis are symptoms familiar to all. Fever is not usual and the illness is over in a few days. Secondary bacterial infection can lead to otitis media, sinusitis or acute bronchitis. In these circumstances either *Strep. pneumoniae* or *H. influenzae* is responsible. and ampicillin is usually effective treatment.

Acute Sore Throat (Pharyngitis and Tonsillitis)

Streptococci and adenoviruses are the usual causes of pharyngitis and tonsillitis. A sore throat can also be part of the symptom complex of infections by influenza, parainfluenza, coxsackie A, ECHO virus and diphtheria, and is a common feature of infectious mononucleosis.

The pharynx is inflamed and an exudate may be seen on the tonsils. A yellow exudate is a regular but not diagnostic feature of a streptococcal sore throat, and is seen also with adenovirus and infectious mononucleosis. The tonsillar lymph nodes often enlarge and become tender. If the nodes in the posterior triangle become enlarged, then infectious mononucleosis should be considered and the presence of petechiae on the palate makes this diagnosis likely. Ulceration of the throat and gums suggests a coxsackie A infection, but a herpes simplex infection occurring for the first time in a young adult can produce ulceration of the pharynx, buccal mucosa and lips. Although immunization has considerably reduced the incidence of diphtheria in developed countries, it should still be considered.

Where there is ulceration or features indicative of infectious mononucleosis, antibiotics can be withheld, but because of the similarity between the streptococcal and the virus sore throat, most physicians would prescribe penicillin or erythromycin for acute exudative tonsillitis associated with fever.

Acute Laryngitis (Croup)

Acute laryngitis occurs frequently in young children and is almost always due to parainfluenza virus. The child has a cough and hoarseness leading to stridor and rib recession. The stridor can come on very quickly, but the rate of spontaneous improvement can also be rapid. The decision regarding admission to hospital is often a difficult one, but any young child with severe or prolonged symptoms, particularly if there is evidence of hypoxaemia such as cyanosis or restlessness, should be admitted. The distinction between croup and epiglottitis can be very difficult and if there is any doubt it is safest to admit the child to hospital. The milder cases can be treated at home and given humidified warm air to help relieve the airway obstruction. This atmosphere can be achieved by nursing the child in the bathroom with the hot tap running. Mild sedation can be given, if necessary, using promethazine syrup.

Children with severe symptoms may need intubation and corticosteroids are often given, but these are of doubtful benefit.

Acute Epiglottitis

Acute epiglottitis is a severe illness with a significant mortality due to respiratory obstruction (25 per cent in one series). It is caused by the type B *H. influenzae* (the capsulated form) and is commonest between the ages of six months and three years.

There are several features which are helpful in distinguishing acute epiglottitis from a virus croup. The respiratory obstruction is generally more rapid in onset and is more severe, and the child is ill and toxic. The voice is quiet and muffled but not hoarse, because the obstruction is above the larynx. The very ill and breathless child may not be able to speak, however, and this sign may not be apparent. The most reliable sign is the appearance of the epiglottis itself. This protrudes above the back of the tongue with a bright cherry-red appearance and is usually obvious with the aid of a tongue depressor, but care is necessary because the use of this instrument may itself precipitate obstruction.

Suspicion of the diagnosis is an indication for immediate admission to hospital where the child can be intubated. Intubation is continued until the acute redness and swelling of the epiglottis has subsided, which usually happens after three days. In the past, ampicillin has been the drug of choice, but where there is known to be a significant local incidence of resistant *Haemophilus*, there is a good case for using chloramphenicol and some of the newer cephalosporin antibiotics look promising. Many physicians give hydrocortisone as well, although the benefit of this treatment is unproven.

Acute Tracheobronchitis

Following a cold or sore throat there may be progression to retrosternal soreness, cough, sputum and wheezing. Respiratory syncytial virus may be responsible in children, but influenza is the likely cause in adults. Some cases are undoubtedly due to mycoplasma pneumoniae, and there may be an element of secondary bacterial infection. If purulent sputum is being produced, then antibiotic treatment is indicated and if wheezing is a prominent symptom, bronchodilators will help.

Acute Bronchiolitis of Infancy

Acute bronchiolitis of infancy is almost always due to respiratory syncytial virus, so-called because it produces a giant cell cytopathic effect. Infants under one year of age are affected, and most are younger than six months old.

The predominant features of bronchiolitis are cough, wheezing and a rapid respiratory rate. There is chest recession, and wheezes and crackles are heard. Visible distension of the chest and increased translucency of the lungs on the chest radiograph are frequent and are of high diagnostic significance. The mildest cases can be treated at home, but most infants are hypoxaemic and should be treated in hospital where there are facilities for nasogastric feeding and administration of oxygen.

Influenza

Virtually all instances of influenza are due to influenza A or B. Influenza is a highly infectious disease, occurring in epidemics as well as being endemic throughout the world. Disease due to influenza A is more severe than B and the A strain is responsible for most epidemics.

With an incubation period of only two days it is common for all members of a family to be ill simultaneously and for a large proportion of groups, such as office staff, to be absent from work at the same time.

The symptoms are mainly those related to a fever and may start abruptly. There is headache, general muscle aching and a variable degree of prostration. Respiratory symptoms can be absent, but a slight cough is usual, and tracheobronchitis is common. In the uncomplicated case the fever settles in three or four days and symptomatic treatment is all that is usually needed.

A wide variety of complications can occur, including a number of neurological syndromes, myocarditis and pericarditis. The main complications, however, relate to the respiratory system, and whilst these can occur in previously healthy individuals, the elderly and those with pre-existing lung disease are at particular risk. Tracheobronchitis is common and sometimes an influenzal pneumonia may occur which is serious and can be fatal. However, postinfluenzal bacterial pneumonia is the commonest form of pneumonia encountered. Staphylococcal pneumonia is the most serious complication and is responsible for many of the deaths in influenza epidemics; this is described elsewhere.

Vaccination against Influenza

Prevention of influenza can be achieved to some extent by vaccines given as killed virus by intramuscular or subcutaneous injection, or as live attenuated virus inoculated intranasally. The degree of protection is variable but is in the order of 50 to 60 per cent. In the UK it is usually recommended for patients with chronic heart or lung disease and is also offered to health workers.

Whooping Cough (Pertussis)

Whooping cough is characterized by paroxysms of coughing followed by a forced inspiratory whoop. At first the illness is similar to a common cold but a cough gradually develops and becomes paroxysmal at the end of the second week. These paroxysms are most frequent at night and they commonly promote vomiting which can be sufficiently frequent to interfere with nutrition. There are often signs of bronchitis and the coughing may cause subconjunctival haemorrhage. A relative lymphocytosis is common and the organism *Bordetella pertussis* can be grown from the postnasal space.

The illness normally lasts for about six weeks, but during subsequent respiratory infections the characteristic cough can return and this tendency can last for some months. Infants can be seriously ill and there is a mortality of about one per cent. Complications include pneumonia, lobar collapse and an encephalopathy.

Erythromycin and ampicillin are only effective if given in the early catarrhal stage of the illness and so treatment is usually supportive with particular care given to feeding and resuscitative measures as necessary.

Immunization with killed vaccine gives good protection against infection. It is usually given in combination with diphtheria and tetanus vaccine. The side-effects of the pertussis vaccine have been exaggerated but have led to a marked reduction in the number of babies being immunized. As a consequence there has been an increase in the incidence of whooping cough.

3. Pneumonia

The great majority of pneumonias are due to infection, but a similar clinical or pathological picture can result from other agents, so that pneumonia can be broadly classified as follows:

1. Infective—bacterial, rickettsial, viral, fungal and protozoal.

2. Allergic—pulmonary eosinophilia due to drug idiosyncrasy, *Ascaris* infestation or bronchopulmonary aspergillosis.

3. Physical—radiation, irritant gases.

4. Chemical—lipoid pneumonia.

Pneumonia can be further classified according to the anatomical distribution of the inflammation, as identified radiographically:

1. Lobar.

2. Segmental.

3. Lobular (bronchopneumonia).

Pneumonia can also be termed:

1. Primary—occurring in patients without pre-existing lung disease or other significant medical condition.

2. Secondary—where there is chronic lung disease or obvious predisposing cause, such as immune suppression, stroke, overdose, hypothermia or prolonged immobility or coma for other reason.

A classification according to the causal agent is also possible, e.g. staphylococcal pneumonia, mycoplasma pneumonia.

Table 1 lists the organisms responsible for most infective pneumonias, excluding tuberculosis.

Table 1. Organisms responsible for pneumonias, excluding tuberculosis.

Bacterial	Mycoplasma	Rickettsial and viral
Streptococcus pneumoniae (pneumococcus)	*Mycoplasma pneumoniae*	*Coxiella burneti* (Q fever)
Staphylococcus pyogenes		Chlamydia psittaci (psittacosis)
Klebsiella pneumoniae (Friedlander's pneumonia)		Influenza A and B
Haemophilus influenzae	Uncommon	Parainfluenza
Pseudomonas aeruginosa		Respiratory syncytial virus
Legionella pneumophila (Legionnaire's disease)		

Pathology

The basic abnormality in pneumonia is an inflammatory reaction in the alveoli, with a cellular exudate into the alveolar spaces (Plate 1). The usual sequence is complete resolution of the exudate, but sometimes there is necrosis of alveolar walls and a lung abscess is formed. This is likely to occur in staphylococcal and Klebsiella infection, and lung necrosis is also a feature of primary influenzal pneumonia.

Clinical Features

The clinical features are very variable, depending not only on the causative agent and on the extent of the pneumonia, but also on such factors as age and the presence of underlying lung disease or systemic disease.

The most constant features are fever and cough. Sputum is usually produced at some stage of the illness, but may be very scanty. It can be mucoid, mucopurulent or purulent, and is frequently bloodstained. Breathlessness is a common feature and may seem to be out of proportion to the extent of the pneumonia. Pleuritic pain occurs particularly in bacterial pneumonias. Delirium is found in severe pneumonia and in the elderly, and in seriously ill patients there may be a clammy skin, cyanosis and jaundice.

The signs in the lungs may be florid with bronchial breathing and bronchophony indicating a lobar consolidation or there may only be scattered crackles as in a lobular pneumonia. At times an area of pneumonia may not be detectable clinically, and radiography may show a segmental consolidation in a clinically 'silent' area, e.g. in the medial segment of the right lower lobe.

Pleural friction is likely to be heard if the patient is seen to 'catch his breath' on inspiration, but is sometimes an obvious sign in the absence of pain.

Herpes simplex is a common finding and is usually a sign of bacterial pneumonia.

The clinical and radiographic features of pneumonia can be common to infection by almost any of the microorganisms, but there are certain features which tend to be more characteristic of certain infections, and make it worthwhile describing them individually.

Pneumococcal Pneumonia

Influenza-like symptoms are common at the beginning of pneumococcal pneumonia and are followed by pleuritic chest pain. Breathlessness follows and there is a painful cough.

The sputum is very variable both in quantity and in appearance. A rust-coloured sputum is characteristic, but it may just be purulent or there may be frank blood.

On examination the patient is often hot and cyanosed with rapid shallow breathing and a tachycardia. Signs of consolidation will be present, usually with a pleural friction rub.

Staphylococcal Pneumonia

Although staphylococcal pneumonia can occur in the absence of any other infection and in completely healthy individuals, it is usual for staphylococcal pneumonia to occur after influenza or where the patient's resistance has been lowered.

The illness is usually severe and there is a high mortality even when appropriate antibiotics are given. Sometimes patients die within a few hours of the onset of symptoms. Thin-walled abscesses are a feature of staphylococcal pneumonia, and it is common for them to rupture through the pleura to give a pyopneumothorax (Plate 2). Permanent lung damage can result from a severe infection with bronchiectasis and cyst formation.

Klebsiella Pneumonia

Elderly debilitated patients are the usual sufferers from Klebsiella pneumonia, and the upper lobe is most often affected. It is common for the area of consolidation to become cavitated and there is bulging of the fissure. It is not a common pneumonia, but it has a high mortality.

Mycoplasma Pneumonia

Mycoplasma pneumoniae is best classified as a small bacterium. It can be cultivated on a cell-free medium, but is slow and difficult to grow.

Mycoplasma pneumonia occurs most commonly in children and young adults, and tends to occur in epidemics every two to three years. It is responsible for between 10 and 40 per cent of cases of pneumonia, depending on whether there is a current epidemic. It is common for several members of a family to be infected, although some may have an upper respiratory infection only.

There are no specific symptoms, but headache can be very prominent. The cough is often unproductive initially, and sputum is only scanty and is either mucoid or has only slight purulence. Pleuritic pain is rare. The radiographic changes are those of a lobar or segmental pneumonia, and more than one lobe can be affected. A more widespread nodular pattern of consolidation is seen in some patients who tend to have a more prolonged illness with a cough continuing for some weeks. In the majority of cases, however, the course is benign and the symptoms settle within two weeks.

The total white blood count is usually not raised but there can be an eosinophilia. Cold agglutinins are found in the blood in about 50 per cent of the patients, but these are not specific to mycoplasma infection. Haemolysis is a well recognized but uncommon complication, and other complications include erythema multiforme and arthritis. The diagnosis is made by demonstrating antibodies in the serum. A single titre of 250 is probably significant, but a fourfold rise in titre is regarded as diagnostic of current infection. Sometimes antibody production is slow, and antibodies may not be demonstrated until the third week of illness.

The organism is sensitive to tetracycline and to erythromycin. It is worth giving tetracycline to the symptomatic patient because a response is often seen, but if the diagnosis is confirmed only when the patient has recovered, no treatment is necessary. Erythromycin is given to children because of the adverse effect of tetracycline on the teeth and to patients with poor renal function because renal failure can be precipitated by tetracycline.

Q Fever

Q fever was first described in 1937 when there was an outbreak of febrile illness amongst meat-packers in Brisbane, Australia. Initially the organism was not detected and it was named 'Q' for query fever. This was later identified as a Rickettsia and is now known as *Coxiella burneti*. It is distributed worldwide in animals, birds and insects, and is thought to be conveyed to domestic animals by ticks and mites. The disease in humans is probably derived mainly from cattle and sheep by the ingestion of infected milk, by inhalation of infected dust or by handling of an infected placenta or carcass. However, *C. burneti* survives well in the environment, which accounts for the high proportion of patients who give no history of contact.

The incidence is difficult to determine because it can cause disease mild enough to escape attention, but surveys of primary pneumonia in the UK indicate that it is responsible for three or four per cent of cases. In most cases there is a pneumonia, but in one series as many as 25 per cent of cases had a non-specific febrile illness.

There is an incubation period of between two and three weeks before the onset of febrile symptoms followed by cough, variable sputum and some pleurisy. The pattern on radiography is not specific, showing either lobar or multisegmental consolidation. The diagnosis is made by the demonstration of complement fixing antibodies in the serum. The organism is sensitive to tetracycline, but clearing of the pneumonia can be quite slow.

The other important manifestation is an endocarditis, and this diagnosis should be considered in any patient thought to have an infective endocarditis in whom the blood cultures are negative.

Psittacosis

Psittacosis is a disease mainly of birds of the parrot family, but other birds, such as pigeons and turkeys, can be infected. The organism involved is Chlamydia psittaci, and humans contract the disease by contact with sick birds. The infected bird is listless with dirty plumage and has a watery green diarrhoea. Organisms are present in the urine and faeces, in secretions from the nostrils and in the feathers. Close contact is not necessary because if the bird flaps its wings there will be airborne spread of the organisms. The incubation period is seven to ten days.

Most human cases are derived from recently imported birds, usually parrots, but in many cases no good history of contact can be obtained.

The clinical picture varies from a mild febrile illness to quite severe prostration. The onset comprises influenza-like symptoms with headache and muscle pains, followed by mild respiratory symptoms, but cough is often not prominent. The radiographic signs are variable with a lobar or segmental consolidation, and sometimes a bilateral lobular pneumonia. The diagnosis is made by the demonstration of a high or rising antibody titre. The organism is sensitive to tetracycline, which is effective if given early in the illness. Often the diagnosis will be retrospective and the patient will have recovered with or without appropriate antibiotics or with no treatment at all.

Legionnaire's Disease

This severe pneumonia derived its name from the epidemic which occurred in Philadelphia, USA, in July 1976 at a meeting of the Pennsylvania branch of the American Legion. There were 183 cases, of whom 16 per cent died.

Legionnaire's disease was subsequently found to be caused by a Gram negative bacterium, *Legionella pneumophila*, and some previous pneumonia epidemics have been shown in retrospect to be due to this organism. Sporadic cases have also been identified and an awareness of the condition may show it to be a regular, if infrequent, pathogen. The source of infection is unknown but it has been isolated from standing water; there is no evidence of person-to-person spread. A short incubation period of two to ten days is followed by fever and pneumonic symptoms with usually lobar consolidation. The most severe illness occurs in patients with pre-existing illness and the major complication is renal failure. The diagnosis is made by demonstrating specific antibodies in the blood, but these usually develop from the third week onwards.

At present erythromycin is regarded as the drug of choice, but its clinical efficacy is difficult to assess. From in vitro and guinea pig studies other antibiotics show efficacy against Legionnaire's bacillus, but more information on these is awaited.

Predisposing Factors in Pneumonia

Although there may be no predisposing factors, pneumonia is more likely to occur in certain circumstances:

1. Chronic lung disease, e.g. chronic bronchitis and bronchiectasis.

2. Exposure to cold, perhaps in association with excess alcohol.

3. Postoperative, particularly after upper abdominal operations.

4. Bronchial obstruction, e.g. partial obstruction by carcinoma, adenoma or foreign body.

5. Virus infection, e.g. influenza. This commonly precedes pneumococcal infection.

6. Defective immunity. Myeloma and chronic lymphatic leukaemia often present as a pneumonia, and pneumonia is prone to occur when immunity has been suppressed by treatment of other diseases, e.g. lymphomas and leukaemias.

7. Prolonged coma, e.g. following stroke or overdose.

8. Dysphagia. Any condition causing dysphagia with resulting aspiration, e.g. oesophageal obstruction, neurological disease.

9. The weak and aged.

10. Heart failure.

Investigation of Pneumonia

Investigation is performed to determine the causative agent and to identify any predisposing factors that may also need attention.

Full investigation is by no means always necessary and facilities are often not immediately available.

Chest Radiograph

Radiography is one investigation that should always be carried out at some stage. It need not be done during the illness if easy access to radiology is not available, but a film four to six weeks after recovery to check that the lungs are clear will help exclude an underlying bronchial obstruction, for example by carcinoma or foreign body.

Ideally a chest radiograph should be obtained at the earliest opportunity and this should be repeated two to three days later to check that resolution is progressing. Further films will be needed if there is deterioration or if a pleural effusion is suspected. Sometimes pleural fluid accumulates early in a pneumonia.

Sputum

Ideally sputum specimens should be collected before antibiotic treatment is instituted, but this is not always possible, because sputum may not be produced for several days.

Gram-stained Smear

Although not widely used this can be helpful in staphylococcal pneumonia when clusters of Gram positive cocci may be seen and also in pneumococcal pneumonia in which Gram positive diplococci are often numerous.

Culture

Prompt transfer of the sputum specimen to the laboratory is important and both aerobic and anaerobic cultures are carried out. The latter are particularly important where the pneumonia has resulted from aspiration, and when there is a complicating lung abscess or empyema.

Interpretation of the results of sputum culture is often difficult, because the bacteria involved can be found as commensals. Pneumococci and *H. influenzae* can be inhabitants of the upper respiratory tract and even staphylococci may not be active as pathogens. Pseudomonas is often grown in patients with chronic lung disease and when previous antibiotic therapy has been given, but only occasionally will it be a pathogen. Similarly, the growth of *E. coli* is usually an indication of previous antibiotics and it is rarely a pathogen.

Most anaerobes are derived from the oropharynx and the growth of an anaerobe may therefore mean that the sputum has been contaminated by saliva. Many physicians in the USA favour the use of transtracheal puncture to avoid this contamination, but this technique is not favoured in the UK.

Blood Culture

The growth of bacteria from the blood is most likely with staphylococcal and pneumococcal pneumonia, but only those patients with a more severe illness tend to have a positive culture.

Culture of Pleural Fluid

Although any fluid aspirated should be cultured for bacteria, it is unusual to grow any bacteria unless the fluid is purulent.

Lung Aspirates

Occasionally it is justified to obtain material by percutaneous lung aspiration, particularly in patients in whom an opportunist infection is suspected, but the technique of alveolar lavage through a flexible bronchoscope is a safer procedure for the patient.

Virology

Whilst it is often possible to make the diagnosis only in retrospect and there may not be any therapeutic implications, illness due to Mycoplasma, Q fever and psittacosis can be identified by these methods and appropriate treatment given.

Throat Swab for Virology

If the illness is of less than five days' duration, a throat swab for virology can be worthwhile. The virus can be demonstrated on tissue culture or, in the case of respiratory syncytial virus, by immunofluorescence.

Serological Tests

Serological tests are the usual methods for making the diagnosis of viral, mycoplasma and rickettsial infections. A fourfold rise in complement fixing antibody is indicative of current infection. A blood sample is taken as early as possible and repeated 10 to 14 days later. Sometimes the antibody production can be delayed and a third sample may be necessary to provide the diagnosis. If the illness is already of more than two weeks' duration, it may be too late to demonstrate rising antibody titres, and interpretation of a single titre has to be made. In general a titre of 250 or above is likely to be significant, but it should be stressed that this could represent previous infection.

White Cell Count

A neutrophil leucocytosis is suggestive of bacterial pneumonia, but this may not develop in the elderly or in those with overwhelming infection. In non-bacterial pneumonias a leucocytosis is less likely and a total white count of more than $15 \times 10^9/l$ is almost always due to a bacterial infection. Apart from a moderate eosinophilia that can occur in mycoplasma infection, the differential white count is usually unremarkable.

Cold Agglutinins

Cold agglutinins are suggestive but not diagnostic of mycoplasma infection. A single high titre occurs in about one half of cases.

Differential Diagnosis of Pneumonia

A wide variety of conditions can cause pulmonary shadowing on the chest radiograph, but in practice the following conditions are most often considered in the differential diagnosis:

1. Pulmonary infarction. The distinction can be very difficult, but an initial high fever and pus in the sputum from the onset are useful indications of a pneumonia. The two conditions can, of course, co-exist.

2. Bronchopulmonary aspergillosis. This should be considered in any asthmatic patient developing a 'pneumonia', and the blood examined for precipitins to *Aspergillus fumigatus*.

3. Pulmonary oedema. This can be confused with diffuse lobular consolidation.

4. Bronchial carcinoma.

5. Tuberculosis.

Complications of Pneumonia

1. Lung abscess (q.v.) is common in staphylococcal and klebsiella infection.

2. Pleural effusion. A serous effusion is common in pneumococcal pneumonia and is usually sterile.

3. Empyema is much less common than formerly, but is still seen. Rupture of a staphylococcal abscess can give a pyopneumothorax.

4. Jaundice is a feature of severe pneumonias. The mechanism is uncertain in many cases.

5. Septicaemia with resulting meningitis, brain or liver abscess and septic arthritis. This is unusual.

6. Lack of resolution. Pneumonia sometimes heals by fibrosis, and there is some evidence that this is a result of the presence of foreign bodies.

Management of Pneumonia

The decision as to whether the patient should be managed at home or in hospital will depend mainly on the severity of the illness, the certainty of diagnosis and the availability of help at home, but later transfer to hospital may be necessary in the event of continuing illness or complications.

General

Analgesia. Headache and muscle pains are best managed with aspirin or paracetamol, but more powerful analgesics are often needed for pleuritic pain. Care is needed to avoid suppressing the respiratory centre and the very potent analgesics, such as pethidine, are best avoided in patients with pre-existing lung disease.

Oxygen. This should be given if the patient is distressed or cyanosed or if there is confusion which could be due to hypoxaemia. The usual precaution of giving a low percentage (24 to 28 per cent) is necessary in patients who have a tendency to hypercapnia, i.e. those with chronic airflow obstruction.

Antibiotics. The microorganisms causing pneumonia tend to be eradicated better by some antibiotics than by others, but when treatment is first initiated the causative organism is rarely known.

The antibiotic given should therefore be chosen on the basis of what infection is most likely, and treatment can be modified later according to further information obtained or on the clinical progress. The antibiotics which are appropriate to the individual causative agents are listed in Table 2, but antibiotic treatment is best planned by considering the following groups of patients.

Table 2. Antibiotics for specific infections

Organism	Antibiotic of choice	Penicillin allergy
Streptococcus pneumoniae (pneumococcus)	Penicillin	Many alternatives, e.g. erythromycin
Staphylococcus pyogenes	Cloxacillin or flucloxacillin	Clindamycin, gentamicin, cephalosporins
Klebsiella pneumoniae	Gentamicin, but there may be other sensitivities	—
Haemophilus influenzae	Ampicillin or amoxycillin	Co-trimoxazole
Pseudomonas aeruginosa	Gentamicin	—
Bacteroides fragilis	Metronidazole or clindamycin	—
Mycoplasma pneumoniae	Erythromycin or tetracyclines	—
Coxiella burneti (Q fever)	Tetracyclines	—
Chlamydia (psittacosis)	Tetracyclines	—
Viruses	No effective drugs	—
Yeasts and fungi	Amphotericin 'B' and/or 5 fluorocytosine	—
Pneumocystis carinii	Co-trimoxazole (high dose) or pentamidine	—

The previously healthy and untreated patient. Pneumococcus is the most likely cause and treatment with penicillin is effective. This is best given intramuscularly in the first instance as 0.5 mega unit of benzyl penicillin six-hourly, changing to oral phenoxymethyl penicillin 250 mg six-hourly after 48 hours, providing a clinical response has started. Pneumococcus is also sensitive to many of the other antibiotics, and ampicillin is the alternative most often used. If the patient is allergic to penicillin, erythromycin 500 mg six-hourly should be used.

If there are any features that are atypical, such as mucoid sputum, or lack of pleurisy in spite of lobar consolidation, particularly if there is a known mycoplasma epidemic, then treatment with tetracycline 500 mg six-hourly would be appropriate. As well as being effective against over 90 per cent of strains of pneumococci, tetracycline is suitable treatment for Q fever and psittacosis.

Erythromycin is the antibiotic of choice in children, in all patients in whom poor renal function is known or suspected, and if there is any suspicion of Legionnaire's disease.

When pneumonia follows influenza, Pneumococcus is the most likely causative organism, but staphylococcal pneumonia is likely to occur in these patients and should be covered in any patient who is seriously ill or deteriorating. It should be assumed that the Staphylococcus is penicillin-resistant whether it has arisen at home or in hospital, and flucloxacillin should be given in addition to penicillin or ampicillin.

Patients with pre-existing lung disease. *Haemophilus influenzae* and pneumococcus are the most likely bacterial pathogens in this group and the chronic bronchitic developing pneumonia should be given ampicillin 500 mg six-hourly, or, if he is allergic to penicillin, cotrimoxazole two tablets twice daily.

Failed treatment. There can be a number of reasons why the patient has not improved and so there are no clear rules as to the course of action to be taken in these circumstances.

The suitability of the antibiotic used should be considered, for example, ampicillin is ineffective in mycoplasma pneumonia. In addition it should be remembered that patients can be less than regular in taking their drugs. Pneumonia secondary to an underlying carcinoma or other bronchial obstruction is likely to be slow to resolve. Persistent illness may indicate the development of a lung abscess or empyema.

The diagnosis of pneumonia should also be questioned, and in particular the possibility of pulmonary infarction, tuberculosis, or the 'pneumonia' of bronchopulmonary aspergillosis should be considered.

Further investigation is therefore needed in any patient who has failed to respond or who is deteriorating.

4. Opportunist Infections

Most of the organisms causing pneumonia are normal commensals in the respiratory tract and so to some extent almost all lung infections can be regarded as opportunistic. The reasons why these organisms become pathogenic are often not known, but it is particularly likely to occur when the body's defences are impaired for any reason. This can happen if there is damage to the lung, such as bronchiectasis or cavitation, or if the upper respiratory tract defences have been bypassed by tracheostomy or intubation. Prolonged broad spectrum antibiotic therapy can also predispose to opportunist infection.

The most serious infections are those occurring when the body's defences are impaired because of systemic disease or its treatment, and it is in these patients that infection with unusual agents may be seen. However, it should be remembered that the patient with immune suppression is more likely to be infected by a common pathogen than by a so-called 'opportunist' organism.

The patients mainly at risk are those on immunosuppressive drugs, such as corticosteroids and cytotoxics, those with myeloproliferative disorders, e.g. leukaemia, and those with lymphomas, particularly Hodgkin's disease. When pulmonary shadowing develops in these conditions, it is often very difficult to determine whether it is due to infection, to involvement by the disease, or to a reaction from cytotoxic drugs.

The organisms causing opportunist infections include *Cryptococcus*, *Candida*, *Aspergillus*, *Pneumocystis* and cytomegalovirus.

Cryptococcosis

The yeast *Cryptococcus neoformans* is distributed worldwide and is particularly associated with soil contaminated by pigeon excreta. It is most often encountered as a subacute meningitis in immunosuppressed patients, and capsulated yeast cells can be found in the cerebrospinal fluid. Involvement of the lungs can occur in healthy subjects but this tends to be associated with other conditions, including chronic lung disease. There can be infiltrative lesions, widespread nodularity or large solitary rounded lesions. The diagnosis can be made by examination of the sputum for *C. neoformans* bodies. Treatment is with amphotericin B alone or in combination with 5 fluorocytosine.

Candidiasis

In the severely debilitated or immunosuppressed patient systemic infection with *Candida* can develop, with involvement of the lungs, urinary tract and heart valves. The lungs are most likely to be colonized if there is pre-existing damage, and white plaques of *Candida* can be seen in the bronchi. Invasion of the lungs giving diffuse consolidation results in severe illness and is often a terminal event.

The diagnosis is difficult to establish because *Candida* is so often found in the sputum of patients who have had antibiotics or who are ill for any reason, as well as in many healthy subjects. Its culture from urine is similarly of doubtful significance, because it can be a contaminant. A repeated heavy growth is of greater significance and it can sometimes be isolated in blood culture. Bronchoscopy will demonstrate the endobronchial plaques and alveolar washings can be taken at the same time. More invasive methods (e.g. lung biopsy) can be helpful, but may not be justified.

The treatment of bronchopulmonary candidiasis is with inhaled nystatin and systemic amphotericin B combined with 5 fluorocytosine.

Aspergillosis

Invasive aspergillosis takes the form of an infiltration or a localized necrosis of lung with cavity formation, and is a serious and often terminal condition. It is seen mainly in immunosuppressed patients and is the least common disease caused by *A. fumigatus*. The others are described in Chapter 5.

Pneumocystis carinii Pneumonia

The prevalence of *Pneumocystis carinii* pneumonia has increased in recent years. It was originally described in malnourished babies but is now mainly seen in patients receiving immunosuppressive treatment following renal transplantation or for cancer. There is some evidence that infection is quite common, but that clinical disease only develops when there is malnutrition or immunosuppression. The organism is thought to be a protozoan and is a cyst about the same size as a red blood cell. There is quite often an associated cytomegalovirus infection.

The main feature is gradually progressive breathlessness and radiologically there is most often ill-defined perihilar shadowing which may have a 'ground glass' appearance or may look very similar to pulmonary oedema.

Only rarely can the cysts be found in the sputum, and diagnosis is usually made by examination of alveolar washings taken at bronchoscopy or of transbronchial or percutaneous lung biopsy specimens.

Treatment with pentamidine is effective, given as a daily intramuscular injection (4 mg/kg) for 14 days. Co-trimoxazole in a dose of four to five tablets given three times a day is also effective, and the 70 per cent response rate compares favourably with pentamidine, but co-trimoxazole is less toxic. Clinical and radiological improvement is to be expected within a week, but if this is not the case, pentamidine can still be used with a good chance of success.

Cytomegalovirus

Infection with cytomegalovirus often occurs in association with *Pneumocystis* and the radiological changes are probably similar.

The diagnosis is made by the demonstration of a significant or rising antibody titre, but since antibody production is often suppressed in these patients it may not be possible to prove the cytomegalovirus infection. At present this is not of great importance since there is no specific treatment.

5. Fungal Diseases

Actinomycosis

Actinomycosis is not a true fungus disease, but is best described in this chapter. The organism usually involved is *Actinomyces israeli*, which is a widely distributed anaerobe and is an obligatory parasite.

The usual form of the disease is an infection of the tissues around the jaws and neck with a tendency to form sinuses. The organism enters the tissues around carious teeth or after tooth extraction. It can also be inhaled and produces lung infection in the form of pneumonia, chronic lung abscess or empyema. When the pleura is involved there may be sinuses in the chest wall, with drainage of pus containing the typical 'sulphur granules'. The clinical picture is usually that of a chronic illness with cough and sputum, weight loss and variable fever. It is not a common condition and unless there are sinuses or obvious cervical lesions it is likely to be mistaken for bronchial carcinoma, empyema or bacterial lung abscess.

The diagnosis can be made by demonstrating the Gram positive branching filaments in the sputum or by examining pus from a sinus, but is sometimes only made histologically after thoracotomy.

Treatment is with penicillin, but the response is often slow and a combined surgical approach will often be needed, particularly where there is an empyema.

The least common form of the disease is intra-abdominal infection.

Histoplasmosis

Histoplasmosis is a disease caused by the fungus *Histoplasma capsulatum*. It lives and develops in soil which has been contaminated by bird and bat excreta, and so derelict buildings used by roosting starlings and caves have been identified as sources of infection. The areas where it is endemic are North, Central and South America and parts of Africa, and cases occurring elsewhere have originally been infected in these areas.

The primary lung infection may be symptomless or may cause an influenza-like illness ('cave fever').

Radiologically this primary infection appears as miliary shadowing in the lungs together with hilar lymph node enlargement. This can resolve completely, but there may be calcification of the lesions during healing, giving scattered nodularity in the lungs and sometimes there can be chronic progressive disease resembling tuberculosis with fibrosis and cavitation. There may be an interval of several years between the primary infection and the onset of clinical disease.

The diagnosis is made by finding the fungus in the sputum. A rising antibody titre can be found in the acute illness and the histoplasmin skin test is an indicator of previous infection.

Amphotericin B may be needed if there is severe illness or if the disease is progressive.

Blastomycosis

Blastomyces dermatidis causes the condition that has been called North American blastomycosis. This term should now be avoided because the condition has since been reported throughout Africa as well.

There is a cough, sputum and low grade fever. The chest radiograph shows patchy consolidation, sometimes with cavitation, and the whole picture can resemble tuberculosis. The mediastinal lymph nodes may be enlarged, skin lesions are common and destructive lesions can occur in bone and kidney.

The fungus can be grown from the sputum or from biopsy material and specific antibodies develop in the serum.

South American blastomycosis is the commonest systemic mycosis in the Latin-American countries and is caused by *Para-coccidioides brasiliensis*. It causes ulceration of the mouth and nose and lesions in the lungs. Lymph nodes, spleen and liver can be involved.

Coccidioidomycosis

Coccidioides immitis is a soil fungus found in the semi-arid regions of the South Western USA and Mexico. In these endemic areas a high proportion of the population becomes infected, but only about 20 per cent develop clinical disease. The clinical picture is of an acute febrile illness with a bronchitis or patchy pneumonia, and sometimes hilar lymph node enlargement. These features usually resolve spontaneously after a few weeks, but there can be progression to pulmonary fibrosis, and systemic spread occurs in a few cases. The organism can be cultured from the sputum and the presence of serum antibodies indicates current disease. The coccidioidin skin tests become positive a few weeks after the initial infection.

Aspergillosis

Aspergillus fungi are widely distributed and are found particularly in soil, grain and decaying vegetation. *A. fumigatus* is the fungus most commonly involved in man, and it causes three types of disease:

Allergic Bronchopulmonary Aspergillosis

This is not an infection. Atopic asthmatic subjects develop a sensitivity to the fungus, resulting in recurrent pulmonary infiltrates and a varying degree of bronchiectasis and fibrosis. Skin tests give a dual reaction, with an immediate wheal and flare (type I reaction) and a late (type III) reaction. Specific IgE is present in the serum and precipitating (IgG) antibodies are found in the majority of cases.

The symptoms are mainly those of the underlying asthma, and sometimes there is an exacerbation of symptoms at the time of development of an eosinophilic pneumonia. This is not necessary, however, and an infiltrate is not uncommonly identified during routine radiography. There may be a history of expectoration of brownish plugs. A proximal sacular bronchiectasis is a very characteristic development and there is some contraction of the upper lobe. In severe cases there can be widespread lung damage giving the picture of patchy lung fibrosis.

Systemic corticosteroids produce rapid clearing of the lung infiltrates and should be given whether or not there is coincident worsening of the asthma. It has been suggested that steroids can prevent lung damage if given prophylactically, but until continuous steroid treatment can be shown to be effective in this regard it is appropriate that the intensity of treatment should be dictated by the severity of the asthma.

Mycetoma (Aspergilloma)

Aspergillus grows in areas of damaged lung to form a fungus ball called a mycetoma. The most frequent site is an area of cavitation resulting from tuberculosis, and the incidence of colonization of these cavities is very high. Previous lung abscess, bronchiectasis and sarcoid are among the other causes of lung disease where a mycetoma can develop and sometimes the bronchiectatic area resulting from allergic bronchopulmonary aspergillosis can be colonized by fungus, so that two types of aspergillus disease can co-exist in a single patient.

Radiographically the mycetoma typically shows as a round or oval shadow partially encircled by a halo of air. Sometimes the fungus infiltrates through bronchiectatic spaces to form a much less well-defined growth and this can appear as a more diffuse shadow on the radiograph.

In many instances the patient will be asymptomatic and efforts to eradicate the fungus are not necessary. Haemoptysis is the commonest symptom and troublesome bleeding is the usual reason for treating the local disease. General ill-health and weight loss sometimes develop and are thought to be due to a type III immunological reaction. Almost all patients have *Aspergillus* precipitins in their blood, but a positive skin test is unusual.

Many types of treatment to eradicate the fungus have been attempted and none has been regularly successful. Resection of the affected lobe is the only certain way of arresting dangerous haemorrhage, but requires careful evaluation of the general condition of the patient. The decision to operate is particularly difficult if there are bilateral mycetomata because of the uncertainty as to which side has been bleeding. If there is a single cavity, then repeated irrigation with antifungal agents through a tube can be successful.

Invasive Aspergillosis

See Chapter 4.

6. Parasitic Infections

Amoebic Lung Abscess

Amoebic dysentery is a widely distributed disease in the tropics. Amoebic hepatitis progressing to amoebic liver abscess occurs in a small percentage. A proportion of liver abscesses will burst through the diaphragm and result in amoebic lung abscess. It is usually possible to demonstrate a direct connection with the liver abscess and the diagnosis can be confirmed by finding *Entamoeba histolytica* in the sputum.

Hydatid Disease

This is due to the dog tapeworm, *Echinococcus granulosus*, which is widespread throughout the world, and inhabits the intestines of dogs, wolves and other canines. It is common in sheep-rearing areas because sheep are the main secondary hosts and while grazing they become infected by dog excreta which contains the ova. The resulting embryos penetrate the intestine and pass to the liver where cysts are formed. The dog becomes infected by eating the sheep's carcass, thus completing the cycle. Man becomes infected through handling dogs and, as in the sheep, the embryos pass to the liver or lung to form cysts.

About 25 per cent of cysts are in the lung and they are often bilateral. These are often quite silent but may result in symptoms if there is mediastinal compression or rupture of the cyst. In the latter instance there may be an allergic reaction with wheezing and urticaria, or a transient pneumonia-like illness with blood-stained sputum, which may contain pieces of membrane from the walls of cysts. A blood eosinophilia is usual at the time of rupture. If the parasites die, then the cyst wall can calcify, although this is more likely to occur in the liver. Treatment is surgical, taking particular care to avoid contaminating the pleura while the cyst is being removed (Plate 3).

Paragonimiasis

Paragonimiasis is caused by a trematode fluke which is commonest in the Far East, but which also occurs in Africa and South America and has a life cycle of snails, crustacea and mammals. Man becomes infected by eating crabs and crayfish. The embryo penetrates the jejunum, traverses the peritoneum and arrives in the lung by passing through the diaphragm and pleura. It matures in the lung resulting in cyst formation and fibrosis. The symptoms are chronic cough and haemoptysis, and ova can be found in the sputum. The radiograph shows multiple cysts up to 2 cm in diameter.

Schistosomiasis (Bilharzia)

Schistosomiasis is an infection of the bladder or bowel, but ova can arrive in the lung and cause obstruction to the pulmonary arteries with the development of pulmonary hypertension.

7. Lung Abscess and Empyema

Lung Abscess

An abscess is the result of necrosis of lung tissue within an area of pneumonia. Abscesses can be single or multiple, depending on the cause, and develop in the following circumstances:

1. *Postpneumonic.* An abscess can follow any bacterial pneumonia but is characteristic of Klebsiella pneumonia when a whole lobe can become excavated, and of staphylococcal pneumonia where there are commonly multiple abscesses. Sometimes multilocular cavitation can be caused by an infection with *Pseudomonas*.

2. *Aspiration* of vomit, food and sputum. The site of the abscess is most commonly the apical segment of the right lower lobe and the axillary part of the posterior segment of the right upper lobe. A number of factors predispose to aspiration lung abscess:
(a) Impaired consciousness, e.g. alcoholic stupor, drug overdose, general anaesthesia.
(b) Dysphagia, e.g. achalasia, carcinoma of oesophagus, neurological causes.
(c) Dental sepsis.

3. *Bronchial obstruction.* This may be a bronchial carcinoma or inhaled foreign body.

4. *Septicaemia.* There can be pyaemic abscesses of lung and other organs in bacterial septicaemia.

The symptoms are similar to those of pneumonia, i.e. fever, cough and purulent sputum and sometimes pleuritic chest pain, but at times there are few symptoms and an abscess may present as a radiological finding. Physical signs depend on the size and position of the abscess.

A radiograph taken in the erect position generally shows a fluid level indicating a communication with the bronchial tree. A very large abscess can have a similar appearance to an empyema with bronchopleural fistula.

5. *Other causes.* There are other causes of a cavitating lesion and the differential diagnosis includes:

1. Tuberculosis.
2. Cavitating primary or secondary carcinoma.
3. Cavitating pulmonary infarct.
4. Fungal infection (see Chapter 5).
5. A fluid level in a pre-existing cyst or bulla.
6. Cavitation of massive fibrosis complicating pneumoconiosis.

Treatment of Lung Abscess

Treatment comprises physiotherapy, antibiotics and attention to the underlying cause. Bronchoscopy is necessary to exclude obstruction of the bronchus if there is suspicion on radiography or if the abscess is not resolving.

The antibiotic given will be governed by bacteria grown in the sputum, but if, as often happens, bacteriology is not helpful, a combination of ampicillin and flucloxacillin can be used. If the sputum is particularly foul or if the response is slow, then anaerobic infection should be considered.

The anaerobes involved are likely to be those derived from the oropharynx and are sensitive to penicillin, but in aspiration lung abscess a significant number of infections are due to the bowel organism *Bacteroides fragilis*, which is resistant to penicillin. A combination of penicillin and metronidazole is therefore appropriate. Clindamycin is also effective, but is not the antibiotic of first choice except where there is penicillin allergy since treatment may need to be prolonged, and pseudomembranous colitis is a hazard.

Resolution can take up to three months, but if it is delayed much longer than this, consideration needs to be given to percutaneous insertion of a drainage tube or to lobectomy. A cavitating carcinoma is often very difficult to exclude.

Empyema

The usual causes of pus in the pleural cavity are as follows:

1. Pneumonia. The incidence of postpneumonic empyema has been reduced by antibiotics, but there are patients in whom empyema seems to occur as part of the initial infection.

2. Lung abscess. Rupture of an abscess is particulary prone to occur in staphylococcal pneumonia and a pyopneumothorax results.

3. Tuberculous empyema (q.v.).

4. Subphrenic abscess. The pleural fluid resulting from pus below the diaphragm is usually serous but empyema results if there is direct communication with the pleural cavity.

5. Trauma—penetrating chest wall injuries; intercostal tubes; bronchopleural fistula after lung resection.

6. Rupture of the oesophagus.

The commonest organisms are staphylococci, pneumococci and anaerobic cocci, although it is not unusual for pathogens to be absent, probably because of previous antibiotics. Where the empyema is secondary to a subphrenic abscess there may be bowel organisms, such as coliforms and the anaerobe bacteroides. Mixed infections are quite common, with both aerobic and anaerobic bacteria being involved.

Clinical Features

The presentation varies according to the underlying cause. Fever, chest pain and weight loss are the most usual symptoms, but an empyema can be relatively silent and can progress to become chronic. In this case the pus becomes encysted and the patient develops chronic ill-health with variable fever.

The radiographic features can be similar to those of a serious pleural effusion, but if the pus is encysted there will be a well circumscribed shadow, which can have the appearance of a solid lesion. If a bronchopleural fistula has developed there will be an air–fluid level in the pleural space and it may not be easy to distinguish it from a lung abscess.

Treatment

Treatment is of course dependent on the cause. In the post-pneumonic empyema repeated aspiration of the fluid, together with systemic and locally instilled antibiotics, can be sufficient but if the pus is thick, it may not be possible to aspirate it and drainage through an intercostal tube is preferable. Instillation of streptokinase helps break down adhesions. In spite of these measures, decortication of the empyema is still sometimes necessary, and is the usual treatment for chronic empyema.

8. Antibiotic Treatment for Respiratory Infections

Penicillin. This is the drug of choice for streptococcal sore throat and pneumococcal respiratory infections. Its activity against other respiratory pathogens is unreliable and the majority of staphylococci are now resistant. It is best given parenterally (i.v. or i.m.) in very ill patients, in a dose of 0.5 to 1 mega unit every six hours. Thereafter and in less severe infections phenoxymethyl-penicillin (penicillin V) is given orally.

Ampicillin and amoxycillin. The antibacterial spectra of these two antibiotics are virtually identical and with regard to respiratory infections they are effective against both streptococci and *H. influenzae.* They are therefore the drugs of choice when bacterial infection is suspected in patients with pre-existing lung disease and in patients with acute epiglottitis. However, there are some resistant strains of *H. influenzae. Staphylococcus* and *Pseudomonas* are usually resistant, and the sensitivity of *Klebsiella* is variable.

Co-trimoxazole. This is a suitable alternative to ampicillin in patients with penicillin sensitivity and is of particular use in patients with chronic lung disease. Co-trimoxazole has the advantage of needing to be given only twice daily, but the disadvantage of not being suitable for intramuscular injection. It is probably now the drug of choice in pneumocystis infection, when it needs to be given in high dosage.

Gentamicin and tobramicin. The broad spectrum of these drugs includes *Pseudomonas, Klebsiella* and *Staphylococcus.* They are ineffective against streptococci and therefore need to be given in combination with penicillin or flucloxacillin to cover these organisms. They are also ineffective against anaerobic organisms including bacteroides. A disadvantage of these aminoglycoside antibiotics is that they are not absorbed from the gut. Particular care is needed in patients with poor renal function and in these circumstances the dose should be adjusted according to the plasma levels.

Cloxacillin and flucloxacillin. These are the drugs of choice for staphylococcal infections and cover other Gram positive cocci such as the pneumococcus. The absorption of flucloxacillin is far superior to that of cloxacillin and is therefore the drug used for oral treatment.

Tetracyclines. These have a broad spectrum and are effective against most pneumococci and *H. influenzae*, as well as mycoplasma, Q fever and psittacosis. They are, however, ineffective against staphylococci. The use of tetracyclines has diminished to some extent with the emergence of some resistant strains of pneumococcus and *H. influenzae*, and they should always be avoided in children and during pregnancy because of the yellow staining of teeth that will occur. They should also be avoided in patients with poor renal function and this group includes many of the elderly.

Erythromycin. A useful and probably underused antibiotic, being effective against pneumococcus and other streptococci in addition to mycoplasma infection. It is also active against many strains of *H. influenzae.* At present it is the drug recommended for Legionnaire's disease.

Clindamycin. The main importance of this drug is its activity against the anaerobe bacteroides and it is therefore indicated in some patients with aspiration pneumonia and lung abscess. It is also a useful antistaphylococcal agent and therefore can be an alternative to flucloxacillin in patients who are allergic to penicillin. The main disadvantage is the development of pseudomembranous colitis, which can be a serious complication.

Cephalosporins. There are a number of cephalosporins and it is difficult to summarize them because their antibacterial spectrum is not identical and because some can be given only by injection. None of them can be regarded as antibiotics of first choice for repiratory infections at present. Nephrotoxicity was a problem with some of the earlier cephalosporins particularly when used with a diuretic but the 'second generation' appear to be safer in this regard. About 10 per cent of patients who are allergic to penicillin will also be allergic to cephalosporins.

Chloramphenicol. The use of chloramphenicol should be restricted to life-threatening respiratory infections such as acute epiglottitis. In other conditions when there is *H. influenzae* resistant to ampicillin, an alternative antibiotic is usually available.

Metronidazole. It is highly active against anaerobic organisms, including *Bacteroides* and Clostridia, and is the drug of first choice for amoebic infections.

Fusidic acid. This is active against most staphylococci and can be used in combination with (Flu) cloxacillin in life-threatening staphylococcal infection.

Antifungal Agents

Nystatin. This is only used locally and its main indication is for monilial infections of the mouth and oesophagus. It can also be used for pulmonary infections with *Aspergillus* when given as an aerosol.

Amphotericin B. This is effective against a wide range of yeasts and fungi. For systemic infections it can only be given intravenously, but it can cause acute reactions such as rigors and vomiting, and it is nephrotoxic. The effect on the kidneys may be reduced by giving an infusion of mannitol before and after each amphotericin dose. Nevertheless, it is the toxic effects that are the limiting factors in its use. The drug is given as as infusion dissolved in five per cent dextrose rather than in saline because of precipitation. An initial test dose of 1 mg given over 30 minutes is followed by increasing doses each day with close monitoring of renal function throughout.

5 Fluorocytosine. This has a narrower spectrum than amphotericin, but has the advantage of low toxicity. Its main use is in the yeast infections caused by *Candida* and *Cryptococcus*, but some of these are primarily resistant and it is usual to give amphotericin as well initially. 5 Fluorocytosine is usually given orally, but an intravenous preparation is available for very ill patients.

Miconazole. This is a recent antifungal drug of the imidazole group and has been used for skin and vaginal infections. It has been used intravenously for some systemic fungus infections for which it is still being evaluated. Other imidazole drugs are also on trial.

9. Pulmonary Tuberculosis

Tuberculosis was described by John Bunyan as 'the captain of all the men of death', and it still remains one of the most important infectious diseases in the world, causing between one and two million deaths each year. It has been estimated that there are about 15 million infectious cases of tuberculosis at any one time, of which between 70 and 80 per cent are in the developing countries. These infectious cases almost all have pulmonary tuberculosis and throughout the world this is the commonest form of the disease, accounting for approximately two-thirds of the total.

It is a common disease in many areas, but the developed countries have experienced a marked decline over the years, because of improved living standards, public health measures and specific chemotherapy. In the UK the numbers have steadied in the last five years with between 9,000 and 10,000 cases being notified each year, a significant proportion of whom are of Asian origin.

Clinical tuberculosis results when the infecting dose of tubercle bacilli is sufficiently large and when there is poor resistance in the host. The majority of people becoming infected do not develop symptomatic disease because they overcome the infection. Until 20 or 30 years ago most people, including those of Western Europe and North America, became infected at some time in their lives, but this proportion has fallen markedly since then in the developed countries because of control of the disease.

The infection may be primary or postprimary. Primary disease is related to the site of entry to the body, e.g. lung, intestine, tonsil, skin, and there is enlargement of the local lymph nodes.

Postprimary disease follows immediately or after a variable delay:

1. Direct progression of the primary lesion to give:
(a) Local disease.
(b) Distant disease as a result of bloodstream spread, e.g. miliary tuberculosis, tuberculous meningitis, and later bone and renal disease.

2. Reactivation. This is the cause of most pulmonary disease, and can occur even when the primary lesion has been quiescent for more than 60 or 70 years.

Bacteriology

The human type of tubercle bacillus (*Mycobacterium tuberculosis*) occurs mainly in man and is usually transmitted by infected sputum.

The bovine type (*M. bovis*) also affects humans, but rarely spreads from man to man. The main hosts are cattle, but many other mammals can be infected, both domestic and wild. In man the disease is usually contracted by drinking the milk of infected cows.

Besides the differences in host and in transmission there are differences in morphology between these two types of tubercle bacilli. The human one is a thin rod which is straight or slightly curved and measures $3 \mu m \times 0.3 \mu m$ (Plate 4) whereas the bovine strain appears straight and stubby. There are no antigenic differences between the two, and this accounts for the cross-reactivity on tuberculin testing and the fact that BCG protects against both.

The organisms are relatively resistant to drying and to such chemicals as phenol, but are highly susceptible to sunlight and ultraviolet light. They are killed by heating for 20 minutes at 60 °C—the principle of pasteurization.

The demonstration of tubercle bacilli is proof of active disease, since they hardly ever occur as commensals.

Staining of the sputum by the Ziehl–Neelsen method is the usual means of demonstrating acid-fast bacilli. If large numbers of sputum smears have to be examined, then fluorescent microscopy has some advantage because of speed.

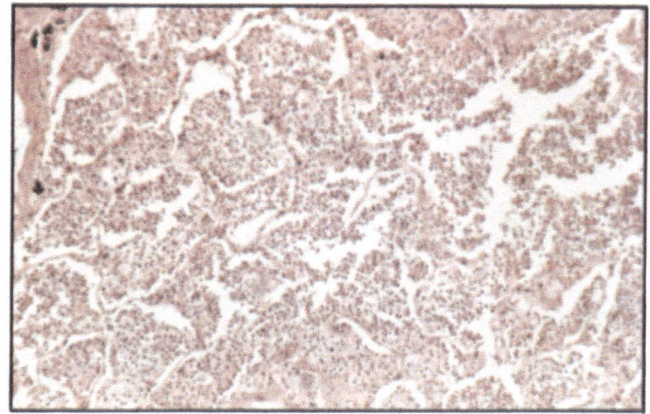

Plate 1. *Lobar pneumonia. Stage of 'grey hepatization' showing alveolar spaces full of polymorphs.*

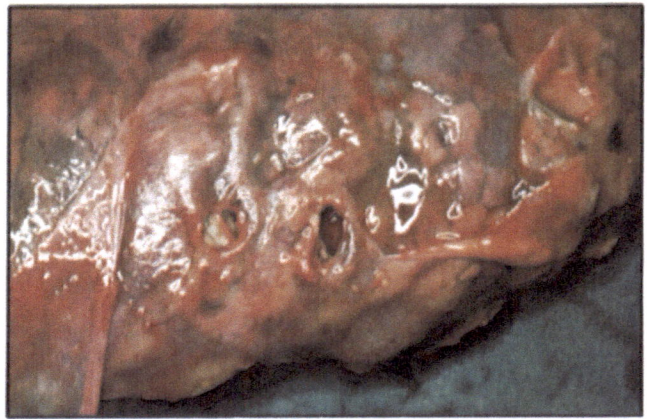

Plate 2. *Staphylococcal pneumonia. Surface of lung showing two abscesses that have ruptured through the visceral pleura.*

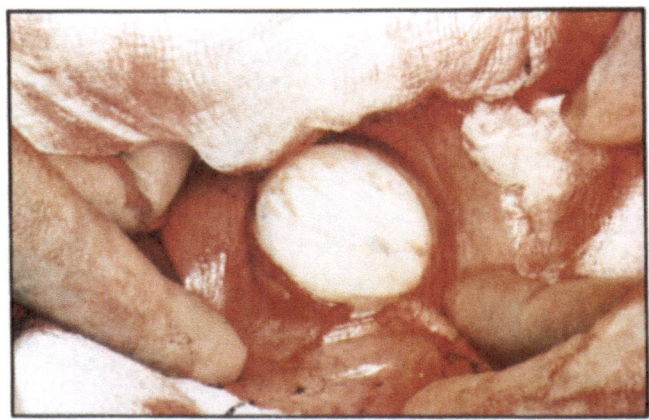

Plate 3. *Hydatid cyst of lung being removed at operation.*

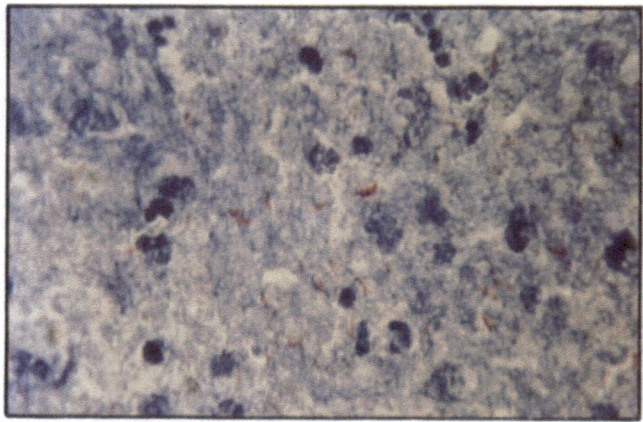

Plate 4. *Ziehl–Nielsen stain showing acid-fast bacilli in pus from cervical lymph node.*

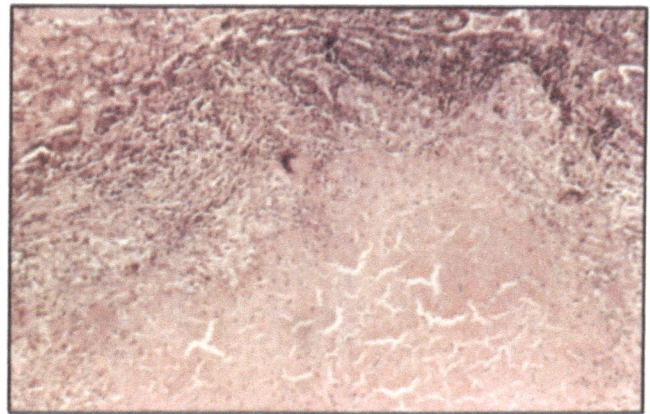

Plate 5. *Chronic fibrocaseous tuberculosis of lung.*

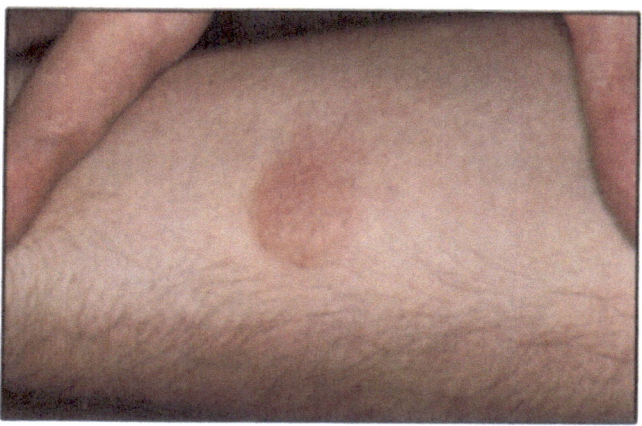

Plate 6. *Heaf test showing grade III reaction.*

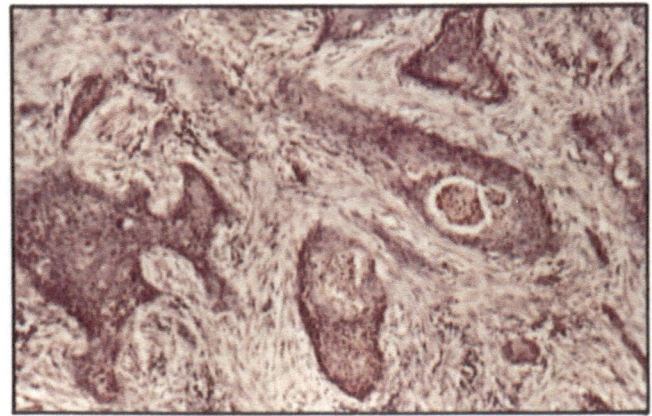

Plate 7. *Squamous carcinoma of lung. Well differentiated. Note typical cell nests with keratinous centres.*

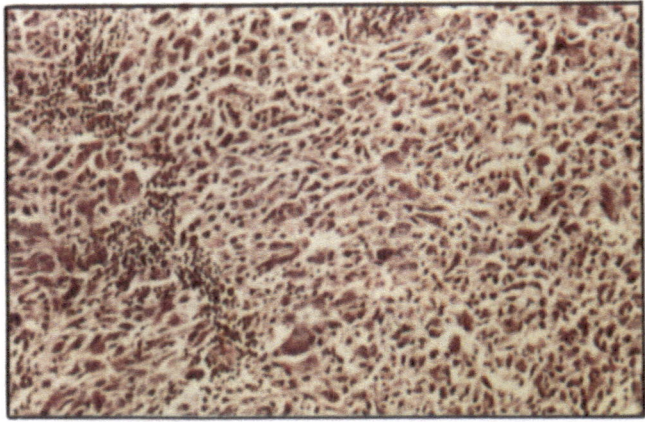

Plate 8. *Anaplastic carcinoma. Predominantly large cell type. Note cellular pleomorphism and lack of differentiation.*

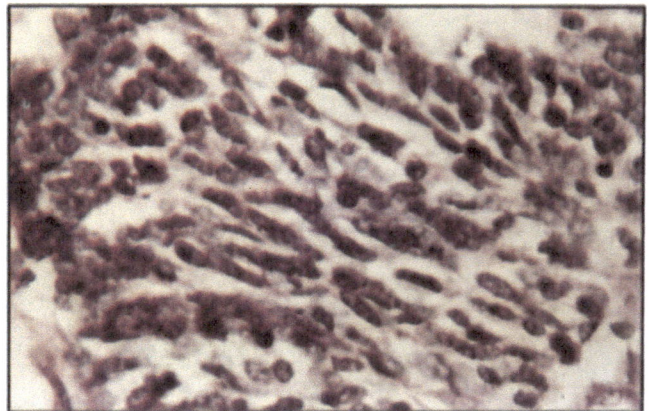

Plate 9. *Oat cell carcinoma.*

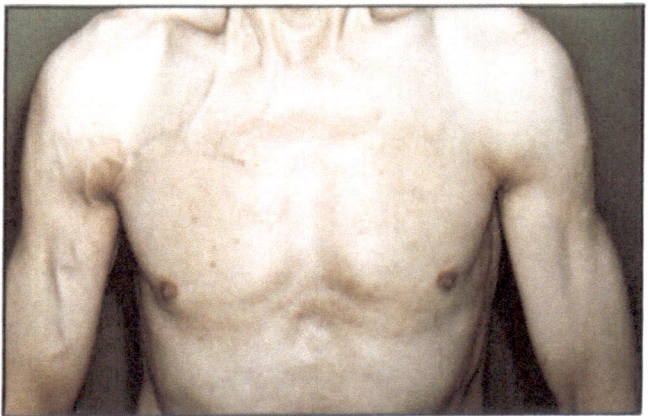

Plate 10. *Superior vena caval obstruction due to bronchial carcinoma showing distension of veins in right shoulder and arm.*

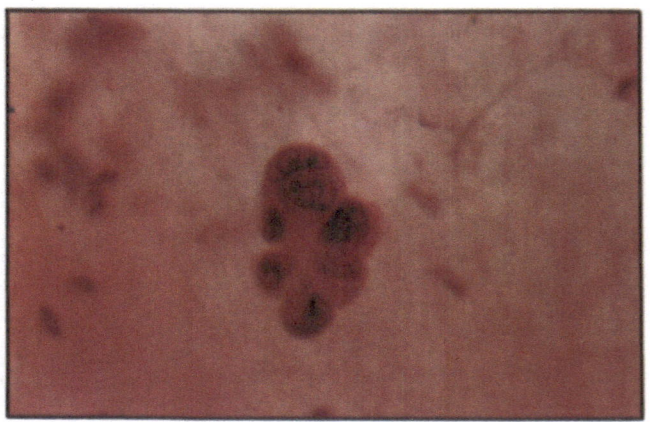

Plate 11. *Sputum cytology showing group of malignant cells from adenocarcinoma of the lung.*

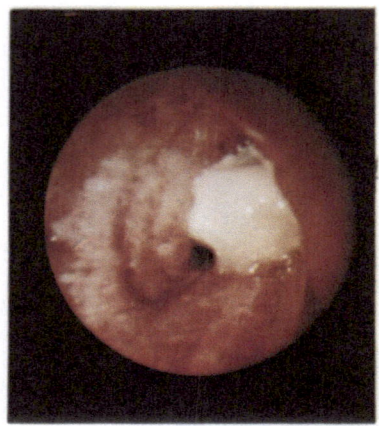

Plate 12. *Necrotic and fungating bronchial carcinoma seen at bronchoscopy. (Courtesy of Dr P. Stradling, Hammersmith Hospital, London.)*

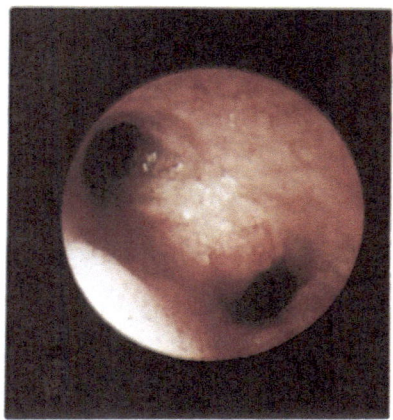

Plate 13. *Bronchoscopic view showing distortion and separation of the orifices of left upper and lower bronchi by enlarged lymph nodes. (Courtesy of Dr P. Stradling, Hammersmith Hospital, London.)*

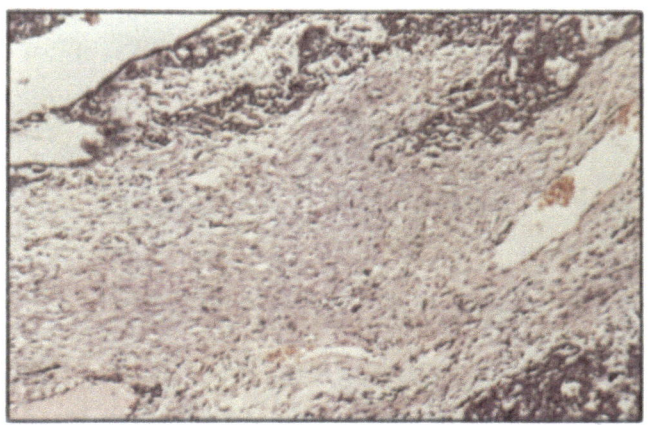

Plate 14. *Mesothelioma of pleura showing fibroblastic (central) and 'glandular' (peripheral) structures.*

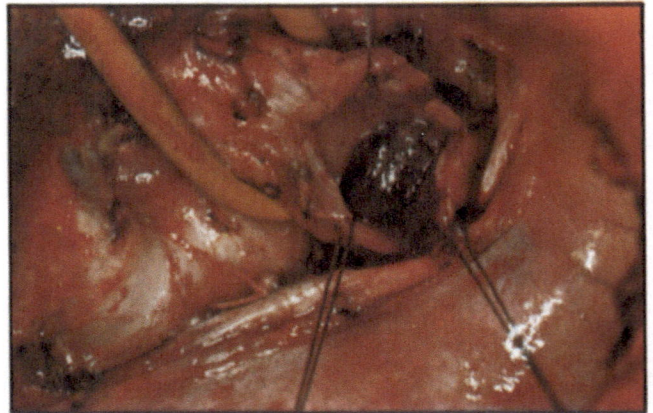

Plate 15. *Bronchial adenoma shown as plum-coloured tumour within the bronchus*

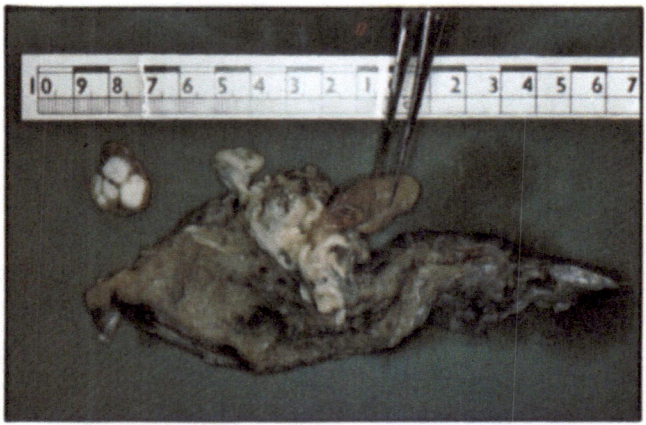

Plate 16. *Hamartoma of lung (held in forceps). The cut surface is shown on the left.*

Final identification can only be made by culturing the organisms or by animal inoculation. An egg-enriched medium, such as Lowenstein–Jensen medium, in screw-cap containers to preserve moisture, is used. Growth is slow, and the earliest appearance is at 10 to 14 days, but is sometimes delayed for eight weeks.

Guinea-pig inoculation may be more sensitive than culture where there are small numbers of bacilli. It is usual to inject two guinea-pigs. One is killed and examined at four weeks or earlier if it has developed any lymph node enlargement, and the other at eight weeks.

Pathology

The basic pathology is of a granulomatous lesion having epithelioid cells, Langhan's giant cells, lymphocytes and a varying degree of fibrosis (Plate 5). There is central caseation, the cheesy form of necrosis, and in later years these caseous areas can become calcified. Tubercle bacilli may be seen in the granulomatous lesions, but their absence by no means excludes tuberculosis.

Conditions Predisposing to Tuberculosis

General ill-health, malnutrition and reduced immunity all increase the susceptibility to tuberculosis, and its increased incidence should be remembered in the following conditions:

1. Diabetes mellitus.
2. Following partial gastrectomy.
3. All patients on corticosteroids.
4. Hodgkin's disease and other lymphomas.
5. Alcoholics.

Methods of Controlling Tuberculosis

The methods available for controlling the disease include the following:

1. Treatment of patients with active disease.
2. Case finding.
3. Control of bovine sources.
4. BCG immunization.
5. Chemoprophylaxis.

Treatment of Active Disease

Pulmonary tuberculosis in man is the most common source of the disease and eradication of tubercle bacilli in these patients plays a major role in tuberculosis control. Patients with drug-resistant bacilli are fortunately not common but are a constant source of infection.

Case Finding

It should be obvious that energetic efforts to detect cases are only useful if the therapeutic services are sufficiently developed to deal with the patients that are identified.

Contact Tracing

The facilities available in developed countries enable household and work contacts to be seen. In many countries these facilities are not available or are not sufficiently developed for this method of control to be employed.

The usual policy is to radiograph all adults and to tuberculin test children. A positive tuberculin test should be followed by a radiograph and in children and adolescents may be an indication for chemoprophylaxis.

Radiography

Mass miniature radiography has played an important part in the past in case finding, but the number of cases revealed by surveying healthy subjects has become too small to make this justifiable on economic grounds. However, this method is still of value in examining selected groups where the yield is likely to be significant. These are as follows:

1. Contacts of known cases.

2. Inmates of lodging houses, institutions for mental sub-normality and prisons.

3. Immigrants, particularly of Asian origin.

In addition to these groups, all patients with persistent respiratory symptoms should have a radiograph taken. There are certain groups of workers who are more likely to disseminate the disease if they contract tuberculosis, and not only should their employment be dependent on a chest radiograph, but they should also be subjected to regular radiographic surveillance, e.g. every two years. The following occupations would be included in this group: doctors, dentists, nurses, schoolteachers and others working with children, hairdressers, and all involved in the preparation or service of food.

Tuberculin Testing (see page 50)

Tuberculin testing can be useful if there is a low rate of tuberculosis within the community and if BCG is not being used, but even then the few with strongly positive tests do not often have clinical disease. The method is unsuitable for routine use, but can give some indication of the current prevalence in a particular community.

Sputum Examination

Examination of the sputum by direct smear for acid-fast bacilli is a useful method for case finding in developing countries where it may not be possible to have and maintain expensive radiography equipment, and where much of the population may reside in inaccessible areas. The cases found by this method are, of course, those who are the most infectious.

Control of Bovine Tuberculosis

Bovine tuberculosis used to be a substantial source of disease in Western Europe, but tuberculin testing of cattle, the slaughter of infected animals and pasteurization of milk has virtually eliminated this source in the UK and USA. In parts of the West of

England tuberculin positive cattle have been reappearing recently and it has been found that the badger population in this area has a high incidence of tuberculosis. Elimination of the badgers in well-defined districts coincided with a reduced incidence of tuberculin positivity in the cattle.

Bacille Calmette Guerin (BCG) Vaccination

BCG vaccine was first developed from the bovine strain whose virulence was modified by its culture on a potato medium. The famous Lubeck disaster in 1930 occurred a few years after its introduction. A large number of infants in Germany died as a result of contamination of the vaccine by virulent tubercle bacilli.

Early trials showed that BCG gave a high degree of protection in North American Indians, and a study of Chicago infants (Rosenthal et al. 1961) in the war years showed 74 per cent protection. A trial of school-leavers in the UK showed a 79 per cent reduction in tuberculosis and a significant degree of protection was maintained for 15 years (British Medical Research Council 1963). In less developed countries the results have been variable, perhaps because of some protection from non-tuberculous mycobacteria, but nevertheless a 62 per cent reduction was demonstrated in South India (Frimodt-Møller et al. 1964).

In Britain it has been standard practice to offer BCG to school-children at the age of 13 years and to nurses and medical students who are tuberculin negative. The routine use of BCG is being discontinued in some areas of Britain as a result of the declining incidence of the disease. In developing countries BCG still provides a cheap and effective means of controlling the disease, but its use is very variable. In those countries where the disease is still prevalent it is logical to administer BCG at birth. 0.1 ml vaccine is injected intradermally at the site of insertion of the deltoid muscle. Local abscess formation may rarely occur and the axillary lymph nodes may swell but serious complications of BCG are very rare. Jet injection techniques have the merit of speed of administration, but produce very variable results.

Chemoprophylaxis

Isoniazid alone is usually given (5 mg/kg/day) but if there is any suspicion of clinical disease a second drug should be given (see 'insurance chemotherapy').

Primary chemoprophylaxis is the administration of isoniazid to individuals who are not infected, but who are at risk, e.g. suckling infants whose mothers are infected. It is possible to vaccinate at the same time by giving isoniazid-resistant BCG.

Secondary chemoprophylaxis is given where there is evidence that an individual has been infected, but has not, as yet, developed clinical disease. There is considerable variation in the practice of chemoprophylaxis between the developed countries themselves as well as the expected variation between the developed and undeveloped countries. In the UK the following should be given prophylactic isoniazid for one year:

1. Subjects who are known to have recently become tuberculin positive.

2. All positive reactors below the age of five years.

3. Child contacts of patients with infectious disease who are tuberculin-positive. The decision here is much less clear-cut, but most physicians would treat children of under 10 years of age.

'Insurance' chemotherapy

Much of the tuberculosis seen in the developed countries results from the reactivation of old and apparently healed disease, and is being seen particularly in the elderly.

Where fibrotic and calcific disease is seen on a chest radiograph and where the patient has not previously had chemotherapy or where previous chemotherapy has been inadequate, a course of 'insurance' chemotherapy should be considered.

It is becoming increasing practice for physicians to prescribe a course of chemotherapy for patients who have radiological evidence of previous disease, but in whom no disease activity can be demonstrated. There is no general agreement on the type of therapy that should be used. In the USA, isoniazid alone is commonly used, but many physicians in the UK are concerned about the use of a single drug and prefer to use a combination of isoniazid and ethambutol for a year or isoniazid and rifampicin for six months. However, trials to determine the optimum duration of treatment with these combined drug regimens are awaited.

Tuberculin Testing

The tuberculin test demonstrates the presence of a type IV (delayed) hypersensitivity. The reaction becomes positive within six weeks of infection. The solution used for tuberculin testing is a purified protein derivative of a culture of tubercle bacilli (PPD).

Mantoux Test

Diluted PPD 0.1 ml solution is injected intradermally into the forearm. It is usual to give 1 tuberculin unit (TU) (1 : 10,000 solution) initially if tuberculosis is likely, and to repeat with 10 TU (1 : 1,000 solution) if negative. A disc of induration of 10 mm or more in diameter is a significant response. It is important that the diameter of induration is measured and recorded in order to aid subsequent interpretation. The reaction is read after two to three days.

Heaf Test (Plate 6)

The multiple puncture test is done with a 'gun' which punctures the skin with six short needles. Undiluted PPD solution (2 mg/ml) is used and is spread onto the forearm to an area corresponding to the size of the round plate of the Heaf gun. The reaction is read at three to six days and is graded as follows:

Grade I   —at least four indurated papules.
Grade II —coalescence of the papules into a ring of induration.
Grade III —a disc of induration.
Grade IV —a larger reaction which may become blistered.

Grades I and II are not regarded as significant since they are not believed to represent previous tuberculous infection, and these patients can be given BCG.

Grades III and IV signify present or past infection.

Tine Test

The Tine test is another multiple puncture test using a disposable unit in which there are four prongs which have been coated with old tuberculin solution. The plastic guard is removed and the prongs are pressed into the forearm. The reaction is read two to three days later, and a positive reaction is indicated by one or more of the resulting papules being 5 mm or more in diameter.

The test is very quick and simple to do, but more information is needed on the comparison with the Mantoux test and with the Heaf test.

Significance of the Positive Tuberculin Test

A positive reaction is indicative of past or present infection or of previous BCG, although the weaker grades of positivity are usually non-specific reactions.

However, the test can be negative in the presence of active disease in certain circumstances. Patients with overwhelming disease, particularly the elderly and those with suppression of their immunity, may have negative reactions. It may therefore be difficult to exclude the disease in patients in whom delayed hypersensitivity is naturally suppressed, e.g. Hodgkin's disease and in those receiving immunosuppressive treatment.

The tuberculin test is of little value as a diagnostic test in adults and its main use is epidemiological, giving an indication of the prevalence of infection within a population.

Clinical Tuberculosis

Primary Tuberculosis

The primary complex consists of the primary lesion together with involvement of the regional lymph nodes. The commonest site of initial infection is the lung, and the primary complex comprises the peripheral lung lesion and enlargement of the draining lymph nodes at the hilum of the lung.

The primary lesion can also occur in the tonsils, causing enlargement of the cervical lymph nodes, or in the small intestine, but these sites are less common now in developed countries because of the decline in bovine tuberculosis.

The Primary Complex in the Lung

The primary lesion is subpleural, and can occur in any lobe of the lung. More than one primary lesion may develop.

Following the formation of a primary complex there may be the following developments:

1. Healing of the primary and lymph node lesions. This is the usual sequel, and there may be subsequent calcification of the primary lesion (the Ghon focus) and of the lymph nodes.

2. The primary focus becomes walled off and the lesion is dormant with a susceptibility to reactivation in later life if the body's defences fail.

3. Local progression of the primary lesion occurs, which can give rise to local cavitation and tuberculous pneumonia, and to tuberculous pleural effusion.

4. Lobar collapse and epituberculosis occur. As a result of the hilar lymph node enlargement there may be sufficient compression of a bronchus to cause collapse of a lobe, particularly of the middle lobe. A valvular obstruction can also occur from the bronchial compression leading to air trapping within a lobe (obstructive emphysema). The term 'epituberculosis' has been used to refer to the area of lobar or segmental lung shadowing associated with the hilar lymph node enlargement. This shadowing is usually a result of a non-tuberculous inflammatory exudate and it can resolve quite quickly, without sequelae. There is at times an element of collapse involved and an actual caseous tuberculous pneumonia, resulting from discharge of a lymph node through the bronchial wall, will give a similar radiological appearance.

Local involvement of the bronchial wall can lead to a stenosis of the bronchus and to permanent lobar or segmental collapse.

Subsequently bronchiectasis in the affected area may occur and presumably this is due to the combination of bronchial obstruction and secondary infection.

5. Haematogenous spread can be either by the pulmonary veins draining a lesion or from the lymph nodes to the thoracic duct and subsequently to the systemic veins.

As a result of haematogenous spread there may be miliary tuberculosis or tuberculous meningitis, both of which usually develop within a year of infection, or disease of bone, kidney, adrenal gland, skin and other tissue, whose occurrence may be delayed. Involvement of the renal tract and of the skin is said to be unusual within five years.

Clinical Features of Primary Tuberculosis

The symptoms and signs of the primary infection are usually few and non-specific and the great majority of patients are asymptomatic. In the event of local spread of infection there may be vague ill-health but respiratory symptoms are often not prominent. There may be physical signs in relation to epituberculosis, and to pleural effusions.

Tuberculous Pleural Effusion

Tuberculous pleural effusion is uncommon below the age of five years. It results either from spread of infection to the pleura from part of the primary complex, in which case it develops within a year of the infection, or it occurs later in life as a complication of postprimary tuberculosis. The development of a tuberculous effusion can be quite silent, but there may be fever and pleuritic pain at the onset. The effusion is often quite large and the fluid is clear and straw-coloured. It is most unusual to be able to find tubercle bacilli in a centrifuged deposit of the fluid, but bacilli may subsequently be isolated by culture. Needle biopsy of the pleura provides the best means of confirmation of the diagnosis and tuberculous granulation tissue is identifiable in over 50 per cent of cases, providing an adequate biopsy has been obtained.

Pleural effusions were formerly a common complication of treatment by artificial pneumothorax, and fibrosis and calcification of the pleura ensued if the effusion was complicated by empyema.

Treatment of a tuberculous effusion. The fluid is aspirated and antituberculous drugs are given. It is standard teaching to give corticosteroids to prevent residual adhesions and pleural thickening, and although there is evidence of their efficacy in this regard, many physicians do not use them routinely, perhaps because therapy is sometimes given in the form of a diagnostic trial.

Miliary Tuberculosis

Widespread dissemination of tubercle bacilli via the bloodstream results in multiple small lesions throughout the body. In areas where tuberculosis is still common, the disease follows primary infection with bacilli being released into the blood from the primary lesion itself or from the caseous hilar lymph nodes. In the developed countries miliary tuberculosis is more often seen in the elderly in whom the diagnosis may be difficult to substantiate.

The young patient is usually acutely ill and pyrexial. The most reliable physical signs are the choroid tubercles, which are yellowish lesions in the fundus less than a quarter of the diameter of the optic disc. The spleen is often enlarged in children. The chest radiograph reveals miliary mottling. These shadows are small (the size of millet seeds) and are evenly distributed throughout the lungs. These lesions are sometimes very difficult to see and the radiograph may be quite normal before they are fully developed.

The diagnosis in the older patient is much more difficult. The disease may be less acute and can take the form of chronic ill-health, with progressive weight loss and low-grade fever. The physical signs of choroid tubercles and splenomegaly are less likely than in children and it is possible for the chest radiograph to be entirely normal. One of the non-specific features of miliary tuberculosis in the elderly is an anaemia, which may be part of a pancytopaenia or there may be a leukaemoid blood picture, together with splenomegaly. A negative tuberculin test does not exclude the diagnosis. Culture of sputum, urine and bone marrow should be initiated, and biopsy of bone marrow and liver may show tuberculous granulomata. In the event of deterioration in the absence of a firm diagnosis, a trial of therapy is justified. The drugs given initially should be those which are specific for tuberculosis so that a response to treatment can be taken as confirmation of the diagnosis. Isoniazid is given together with PAS or ethambutol and a fall in the fever should be expected within two weeks. If the patient is desperately ill and no diagnosis has been obtained, it is justifiable to give corticosteroids as well as initiating standard antituberculosis therapy.

Postprimary Pulmonary Tuberculosis

Since the lung is the commonest site for primary infection it is to be expected that postprimary disease is most usual in the lung.

It arises as a result either of direct progression of the primary lesion, as already outlined, or of reactivation of a quiescent lesion. Reactivation can occur after any interval and is the usual cause of the active disease as seen in the elderly, and in those whose immunity is impaired.

Pathology

The lesions of postprimary tuberculosis occur most commonly in the upper half of the lungs, and tend to be in the posterior segment of the upper lobes. The apical segment of the lower lobe is also a common site. The reason for this distribution is probably related to the reduced blood flow to the upper parts of the lobes compared with the lower parts.

The histological features are those already described. Caseation may be very extensive and the resulting cavitation can be very large. The lesions tend to heal by fibrosis and later by calcifying, but successful chemotherapy appears to reduce the amount of fibrous tissue which forms. In untreated patients whose disease is longstanding, there may be areas of fibrosis and calcification co-existing with active caseating disease.

Symptoms

Small areas of disease are often quite symptomless, and are identified by routine chest radiography.

The following symptoms may be present and their prominence will depend on the extent of disease. The development of symptoms is usually gradual.

1. Cough. There is nothing specific about the cough and, as in carcinoma of the bronchus, there may be an increase in the patient's 'normal' smoker's cough. Initially the cough may be dry, but later there is mucoid or mucopurulent sputum. When cavitation occurs the sputum is often purulent, but the appearance of the sputum is not a very reliable indication of the extent of the disease.

2. Haemoptysis. This varies from blood-streaking of the sputum to obvious frank blood, and occasionally there can be massive exsanguinating haemorrhage, particularly when large cavities are present. The occurrence of haemorrhage in patients whose fibrocalcific disease appears to have healed may be due to bronchiectasis or to secondary colonization by *Aspergillus* to form a mycetoma, and is not necessarily an indication of reactivation.

3. Weight loss. Tuberculosis should always be thought of in patients who are losing weight, and this symptom is often accompanied by other non-specific symptoms.

4. Tiredness, malaise and fever. These are the symptoms of many chronic debilitating diseases and although night sweats are a classical symptom, they can result from any febrile illness.

Signs

The physical signs are often very few. The patient may appear healthy and examination of the chest can be entirely normal even though quite extensive disease is seen on the radiograph. The signs are usually most florid where there has been a lot of fibrosis and contraction of the upper lobes, and the trachea may then be found to be deviated, and there is impairment of percussion over the clavicles. Bronchial breathing is then a common sign, resulting partly from the fibrosis itself, but also due to the main bronchi being drawn upwards to lie nearer the stethoscope. Percussion of the clavicle is always an important manoeuvre, because impairment may be the only physical sign of apical disease. The specific signs resulting from cavities have been passed down over the generations, but they are, to say the least, unreliable.

Diagnosis

Radiology

PA Chest radiograph. Whenever there is persistent consolidation on the radiograph, both tuberculosis and underlying carcinoma need to be considered. The features most characteristic of tuberculosis are patchy, sometimes nodular, shadowing, which lies posteriorly in the upper zones and less commonly in the apex of the lower lobe. Bilateral shadowing in the upper zone is particularly characteristic of tuberculosis. Cavitation within the consolidation may be single or multiple and may be bilateral. A single cavity may be difficult to distinguish from a cavitating bronchial carcinoma or chronic lung abscess. Enlarged lymph nodes at the hilum are common in Asians, particularly young adults, but except in primary disease of children, they are not a feature in the Caucasian population.

Fibrosis and contraction of the upper lobes develops during natural healing and is most likely to develop from tuberculosis, although bronchopulmonary aspergillosis can give very similar radiological appearances. There are other conditions that can give upper lobe fibrosis, but the presence of calcification makes tuberculosis most likely. Considerable calcification of the pleura can result from tuberculous effusion and empyema.

The single rounded lesion (tuberculoma) often produces

difficulties in diagnosis and in management. The presence of calcification does not exclude squamous cell carcinoma or a hamartoma. Concentric increase in size of such a lesion is never due to tuberculosis.

Special views. A lateral radiograph is useful because shadowing may then be seen to lie posteriorly.

Apical views may be helpful in revealing a small amount of shadowing which is obscured by the clavicles.

Tomography is useful for the detection of cavities, but its main diagnostic use is probably for the demonstration of satellite lesions near an apparently single lesion, thereby making tuberculosis the likely diagnosis. The amount of disease seen on tomograms is regularly more than is seen on a plain film.

It is not possible to determine from radiographs whether an area of tuberculosis is active, and terms such as 'no evidence of activity seen' on radiography reports should be avoided since they can give a false sense of security.

Sputum

In cases of suspected tuberculosis at least three sputum specimens should be examined for acid fast bacilli by direct smear and by culture. Early morning specimens are preferable and the assistance of a physiotherapist may be necessary. The results of culture are available in four to eight weeks. Drug sensitivity tests should be done if the culture is positive, and these take another three weeks.

Examination of sputum by direct smear is the cheapest way of establishing the diagnosis and is therefore used widely for case-finding in underdeveloped countries.

Gastric Washings

Where no sputum can be obtained, but the radiographic appearances are suggestive of tuberculosis, gastric washings should be obtained, and the resting juice examined by direct smear and culture.

Laryngeal swabs may yield tubercle bacilli on culture.

Bronchial Aspirates

The aspirates from the bronchial tree should be examined for acid-fast bacilli in any case where the cause of pulmonary shadowing is obscure and diagnostic bronchoscopy is undertaken.

Biopsy

Tissue can be obtained for histology and culture by percutaneous needle biopsy, and this is justifiable in difficult cases, particularly when another disease, such as lymphoma, is known to be present.

Transbronchial biopsy using a flexible bronchoscope can also be used, but the specimen obtained is smaller.

The isolated nodule always produces difficulties, and the diagnosis is often obtained after the lesion has been resected.

Treatment

Admission to Hospital

It is usual practice in the UK to admit patients to hospital for the initial weeks of chemotherapy if they are smear positive, and if there are any social factors which might lead to poor compliance with regard to drug taking. In fact these patients may already have been admitted in order to establish the diagnosis. Evidence suggests that patients rapidly become non-infectious once effective chemotherapy has been started, but many physicians feel that closely supervised therapy in the early weeks, together with the opportunity for patients to discuss their condition further, makes initial treatment in hospital of value.

Chemotherapy

The two main principles of the drug treatment are:

1. That at least two drugs, to which the patient's bacilli are sensitive, should be given together.

2. That the duration of treatment should be adequate.

It is usual to give three drugs initially and when the sensitivities are known after eight to ten weeks, treatment is continued with two drugs. The total duration of treatment will depend on the drugs used, and also on the extent of disease.

Triple Therapy

For many years the combination of streptomycin, isoniazid (INH) and para-aminosalicylic acid (PAS) was the standard triple therapy with continuous therapy lasting at least 18 months. The introduction of rifampicin and ethambutol has enabled PAS, which was the cause of much gastrointestinal upset, to be dropped, and in the UK the following regimens are most often used.

Rifampicin (450 to 600 mg), isoniazid (300 mg) and ethambutol (15 mg/kg) or rifampicin, isoniazid and streptomycin (0.75 to 1.0 g daily) are recommended. After two months, or when the sensitivity results are available, one of the drugs is discontinued. Studies of duration of therapy have shown that nine months of rifampicin and isoniazid is effective, and most physicians therefore drop the ethambutol or the streptomycin from the combinations above after two months. This regimen is well tolerated and is highly effective with 85 per cent of the patients becoming sputum-negative by three months. The rifampicin and isoniazid can conveniently be given in a combined preparation as two tablets every morning.

If the rifampicin is stopped for any reason and treatment continued with isoniazid and ethambutol, then it should be continued for at least eighteen months.

Assessment and Supervision of Treatment

First of all the patient should be reassured that the disease is curable, but that in order to achieve this there must be absolute cooperation. It is of the greatest importance that patients should understand that the drug treatment needs to be continuous, and they often need to be reminded of this. They should also be given an estimate of the intended duration of drug therapy.

Once treatment has been initiated, it is useful to have a routine to follow for subsequent assessment, but flexibility obviously needs to be retained. If treatment has been started as an out-patient, it is useful to make an early assessment at, say, two weeks in order to check that the drug treatment is established and to give the patient an opportunity for discussion. Otherwise it is convenient to assess the patient at one, two, five and nine months. Apart from checking for compliance with medication, the patient is weighed and radiographed. At two months the ethambutol is stopped and treatment continued thereafter with rifampicin and isoniazid. After completion of therapy it has always been traditional to follow the patient at intervals, but a two year follow-up is the most that is needed, and even this is probably not necessary if the patient's compliance has been good and there has been satisfactory resolution on radiography.

Alternative Regimens

Twice-weekly streptomycin (1.0 g) and large doses of isoniazid (15 mg/kg) together with pyridoxine given to outpatients has been shown to be an effective maintenance regimen suitable for patients who cannot be relied on to supervise their own therapy.

In underdeveloped countries the cost and availability of drugs have resulted in a number of alternative regimens being used. The above regimen with the initial use of PAS is useful, and a combination of streptomycin, isoniazid and thiacetazone has given good results in East African trials (East African/British Medical Research Council 1973). Supervision of drug therapy is of particular importance, but this does not necessarily mean the use of medical personnel. The high incidence of drug resistance has been caused by inadequate and unsupervised treatment in the past.

'Insurance' Chemotherapy

This is a form of chemoprophylaxis where the disease is thought to be inactive, but where adequate chemotherapy has never been given. Two regimens commonly used are rifampicin and isoniazid for six to nine months, or ethambutol and isoniazid for one year.

Drug Resistance

The incidence of primary resistance to streptomycin and isoniazid is low (five per cent) and resistance to rifampicin and ethambutol is rare, so that an alternative regimen in the event of resistance to a simple drug is not usually difficult to find.

The main problems arise as a result of secondary resistance in patients who have had treatment which has not been long enough or who have taken their drugs irregularly. Here it is not unusual for multiple drug resistance to occur and there can be considerable difficulty in formulating a suitable regimen. If drug resistance seems likely from the initial assessment, it is sometimes wise to use four or five drugs, pending sensitivity tests, to avoid further resistance developing.

Adverse Drug Reactions

These were common when the old triple therapy was used and a rash and fever developed as an allergic reaction to either streptomycin or PAS in about 15 per cent of patients. Sometimes there was evidence of liver dysfunction, particularly if the drug was not stopped. It used to be necessary to stop all drugs, and then to challenge the patient with each drug in turn (starting with isoniazid) in order to identify the offending drug. The patient was then desensitized to the drug by giving it initially in a very small dose and then doubling the dose each day, or it was reintroduced under corticosteroid cover.

Now that PAS is little used, this sort of reaction is mainly due to streptomycin and is managed simply by changing the drug, usually to ethambutol.

The other drug reactions are described with the individual drugs.

Anti-tuberculous Drugs

Streptomycin

Dose: 1.0 g   intramuscularly daily   <40 years
         0.75 g intramuscularly daily   >40 years

These doses are reduced if renal function is poor, but if possible an alternative drug is used. The drug is best avoided in elderly patients (over 60 years).

Toxicity Allergic reactions, such as rash and fever. VIII nerve damage: giddiness results from damage to the vestibular division of VIII nerve, and can be permanent, but can be avoided if the above doses are not exceeded.

Isoniazid

Dose: 200 to 300 mg orally daily (approximately 5 mg/kg) in a single dose.

Toxicity. This is not common and the drug is normally well tolerated. Peripheral neuropathy can occur in patients who acetylate the drug slowly. Oral pyridoxine 10 mg daily will prevent this complication, but unless the patient is an alcoholic, it is probably not necessary to use pyridoxine routinely.

Liver dysfunction, as a hepatitis-like syndrome, appears to occur more commonly in the USA than in Europe. The difficulties of distinguishing this reaction from infective hepatitis make its incidence difficult to determine.

Rifampicin

Dose: 450 or 600 mg orally daily, depending on whether the patient weighs less or more than 50 kg. Patients should be warned that their urine will become red.

Toxicity. Rifampicin can be toxic to the liver, but this is rare. Transient rises in the liver enzymes are quite common but do not require the drug to be stopped. Close monitoring of liver function is not needed, but a baseline measurement prior to therapy can be useful. It is best to avoid rifampicin in patients who have pre-existing liver disease.

Ethambutol

Dose: 15 mg/kg orally daily (100 mg and 400 mg strength tablets).

Toxicity. Retrobulbar neuritis was recorded in some patients when doses of 25 mg/kg were given, but is very unusual at 15 mg/kg/day. Monitoring of visual fields is not necessary, but any visual symptoms such as disturbance of colour vision should cause the drug to be stopped pending ophthalmic examination. This complication is reversible.

PAS

Dose: 12 g daily orally in divided doses.

Toxicity. The upper gastrointestinal symptoms, including nausea. anorexia and vomiting, make this a very unpalatable drug, which is marginally improved by the use of flavoured preparations.

The hypersensitivity reactions of rash, fever and jaundice occur in 15 per cent of patients.

Thiacetazone

Dose: 150 mg orally daily.

Toxicity. Nausea, vomiting, rash, jaundice and agranulocytosis may occur. British and Chinese populations are particularly prone to develop toxic symptoms and this has limited the use of thiacetazone.

Pyrazinamide

Dose: 40 mg/kg daily in divided doses.

Hepatotoxicity is the major hazard, but hyperuricaemia can also occur.

Prothionamide

Dose: 0.75 mg to 1 g daily orally in divided doses.

Nausea is the main problem and the dose may need to be reduced. Liver toxicity may occur.

Cycloserine

Dose: 0.75 to 1 g daily orally in divided doses.

This is a comparatively weak drug and its main use is to prevent drug resistance developing.

Epilepsy, mental confusion and depression are the main side effects.

Capreomycin

Dose: 1 g daily intramuscularly.

This can be nephrotoxic and, as with streptomycin, damage to the VIII nerve can occur.

Complications of Tuberculosis

1. Cor pulmonale and chronic respiratory failure can develop in later years when there has been extensive lung damage, particularly when there has been surgical intervention, such as thoracoplasty.

2. Mycetoma. Residual cavities and bronchiectatic areas can be colonized by the fungus *A. fumigatus* and a fungus ball (mycetoma) can be formed. Sometimes the fungus is less circumscribed and infiltrates through the air spaces to the damaged area of lung. The presence of a mycetoma is usually revealed as a result of haemoptysis, and it is the prominence of this symptom which dictates whether the complication should be treated surgically.

3. Carcinoma of the lung. Most pathologists recognize the 'scar cancer' arising in an area of lung that has been the site of previous damage, often by tuberculosis.

4. Amyloid. When there is chronic suppuration, such as can occur with fibrocaseous disease and empyema, amyloid disease may develop and present as renal failure, liver failure or diarrhoea, depending on the organs involved.

5. Addison's disease. Tuberculosis remains one of the important causes of hypoadrenalism. This complication should be borne in mind in any patient who has had or is at present suffering from tuberculosis when there is vague ill-health and weight loss.

Infection due to 'Atypical' Mycobacteria

The 'atypical' Mycobacteria have been classified according to their characteristics on culture. They are responsible for between one and two per cent of cases of tuberculosis in humans, and the most important in pulmonary disease is *M. kansasii*. Most isolations are made from men in middle age or older, and a 'dusty' occupation seems to be a predisposing factor. It may be difficult to establish whether the organism is pathogenic in an individual patient because, unlike *M. tuberculosis*, it can be isolated from the sputum in subjects who are free of disease. It is important that compatible radiological change is present before treatment is started.

M. kansasii tends to be resistant to antituberculous drugs, and the choice of therapy may be restricted. In the event of a poor clinical response it is sometimes best for the area of disease to be resected.

M. avium, M. xenopi and *M. intracellulare* can also cause pulmonary disease and the latter, as well as *M. scrofulaceum*, can cause lymph node disease.

TUMOURS

10. Carcinoma of the Bronchus

Since the First World War there has been a remarkable increase in the incidence of bronchial carcinoma. This increase has been mainly in males because of the difference in smoking habits between males and females, but in recent years there has been an obvious increase in females, causing the ratio of male to female cases to decrease from 5.7 to 1 in 1951 to 4.6 to 1 in 1970, and now to around 3.5 to 1. It was during the Second World War that women took up cigarette smoking and this is the likely reason for the increase of cancer in the 1970s. Although there have been improvements in diagnosis and increased awareness of bronchial carcinoma, these factors do not contribute much to the startling change in incidence.

In the UK in 1928 there were approximately 3,000 deaths from respiratory tract cancer, and by 1972 this had increased to 32,000. In the USA there has been an increase from about 4,000 in 1930 to 70,000 in 1971. This trend has been similar in all of the industrialized countries in the last 40 years or so, but has been less apparent in African, Asian and South American countries. The figures for these areas are much less complete, however, and future analysis may reveal similar trends.

The highest incidence is in the urban areas of the industrialized countries, and in both the UK and the USA it is commonest in the lower social classes. Almost one in 10 deaths in all males is now due to lung cancer.

Tumours

Aetiology

Cigarette Smoking

Evidence of the risk of smoking was first provided in 1952 by the retrospective studies by Doll and Hill (1952) of patients with lung cancer, and subsequent prospective studies confirmed the high risk for cigarette smokers. Pipe smokers were much less at risk, but nevertheless fared worse than non-smokers.

It is established that squamous cell carcinoma and small cell carcinoma are closely related to cigarette smoking and the risk increases with the intensity and duration of smoking. Heavy smokers have been calculated to have 30 times the risk of non-smokers and the risk in light smokers is increased 10-fold.

It is reassuring to know that if smoking is stopped the risk is reduced markedly and 10 years after giving up smoking is similar to that in non-smokers.

Occupation

Asbestos. Although mesothelioma of the pleura is the tumour usually associated with asbestos, patients with asbestosis (lung fibrosis resulting from asbestos exposure) have a high risk of developing lung cancer, particularly adenocarcinoma, and this risk is increased by 20 times in cigarette smokers, making it the likely cause of death in this group of workers. The development of asbestosis requires heavy and prolonged exposure and so it needs more than 20 years in the asbestos industry before lung cancer is a hazard. Carcinomas are mainly in the lower lobes, where the changes of asbestosis are most marked.

There have been suggestions that exposure to asbestos may result in an increased risk of lung cancer without asbestosis being present, but there is as yet no proof of this.

The asbestosis hazard ought now to be reduced by public awareness of its dangers and by the regulations regarding protection of asbestos workers that have been introduced in most countries over the last 10 years.

Radiation associated with mining. Inhalation of radioactive gases and droplets can result in bronchial carcinoma and this hazard is encountered in certain types of mining, such as uranium and fluorspar.

Occupational lung cancer was first described from the mining areas in the mountains between Czechoslovakia and Saxony, and the minerals mined by both the Joachimstal and Schneeberg miners contain many radioactive elements. There was an average latent period of 17 years between first entry to the mines and development of cancer.

Subsequently occupational lung cancer has been found in uranium miners in Colorado, and fluorspar miners in Newfoundland. As yet no increase has been reported in uranium miners elsewhere, but perhaps the latent period has not yet elapsed.

Workers in the chromate and chrome-pigment industries have an increased incidence of bronchial carcinoma as have those involved in refining nickel by the nickel carbonyl process. The actual carcinogens are not known. Gas retort workers and those exposed to inorganic arsenicals are other groups of workers at risk.

Atmospheric pollution. The higher mortality in urban areas suggests that air pollution is important, particularly as this factor seems to be acting independently of cigarette consumption. At present it is not possible to define particular carcinogens at fault.

Pathology

Bronchial metaplasia can precede the development of squamous carcinoma. There is a close association between the histological appearances of the bronchial epithelium and cigarette smoking where, in addition to squamous metaplasia, there is basal cell hyperplasia and stratification of the epithelium. A small percentage of smokers have carcinoma in situ.

About 50 per cent of the tumours are central and the rest are peripheral. The central tumours arise as a warty growth in the wall of a proximal bronchus and invade through to the lumen and encircle the bronchus, thus causing obstruction of the bronchus at an early stage. Peripheral tumours are less likely to cause obstruction. They invade and compress lung tissue and not infrequently seem to develop in relation to scar tissue.

Histological Types

There are four main histological types, the proportions of which vary among the published series (Bryson and Spencer 1951; Nicholson et al. 1957; Caplin 1972), and so the percentage incidence given must only be approximate.

Squamous Cell (Epidermoid) Carcinoma (Plate 7)

About 50 per cent of carcinomas are of this histological type. Two-thirds of them are in a large bronchus and they form a large proportion of the central growths. They are often very slow growing, and it has been calculated that by the time of diagnosis the tumour has already been growing for about eight years. It is the tumour most likely to cavitate and it can sometimes calcify.

Undifferentiated Large Cell Carcinoma (Plate 8)

The histological criteria used are variable and so an accurate assessment of the incidence of undifferentiated large cell carcinoma is difficult. The majority seem to be anaplastic squamous cell carcinomas in which the characteristic features of squamous cells have been lost.

Undifferentiated Small Cell Carcinoma (Oat Cell) (Plate 9)

Oat Cell carcinomas account for about one-third of carcinomas, and are characterized by rapid growth and early metastases with death within six months of diagnosis. Four-fifths of these carcinomas are in the larger central bronchi. A histological similarity to bronchial carcinoid tumours has been noted.

Adenocarcinomas

Adenocarcinomas make up 10 to 20 per cent of all bronchial carcinomas, but the incidence seems to be increasing. Most of them occur in the periphery of the lung, and because of their position and the slow rate of growth they can reach a considerable size by the time of diagnosis or they may present with metastases. Although they tend to be slower growing than squamous carcinomas, the prognosis of the latter is usually better, particularly when they are central in origin, because they cause symptoms earlier.

Blood Supply

Blood supply of tumours is usually via the bronchial arteries. Examination of the small pulmonary arteries within the same lobe sometimes shows intimal fibrosis, perhaps due to alterations in blood flow resulting from bronchopulmonary anastomoses.

Spread of Tumours

Tumour spread is direct, lymphatic or via the blood-stream.

Direct spread is through and around the bronchus of origin and directly to the adjacent lymph nodes, the pericardium and the pulmonary veins. More peripheral tumours can invade the pleura and chest wall, intercostal nerves, the brachial plexus, the sympathetic chain and ganglia at the root of the neck, the diaphragm and the vertebral bodies.

By the time of diagnosis, almost all oat cell tumours and about one-third of squamous carcinomas will have spread to the lymphatic system, and at postmortem hilar lymph node enlargement is present whatever the histology in virtually all of them. Spread is usually from one group of nodes to another, but tumours can 'skip' a group. In 10 per cent of cases there is spread from one side to the other, particularly from left to right via the subcarinal nodes. Upward spread to the supraclavicular lymph nodes is common, but involvement of the axillary nodes occurs only if the chest wall has been invaded.

The lymphatic vessels within the lung can become permeated by tumour cells and the resulting condition is known as lymphangitis carcinomatosa. This is not restricted to tumours of the lung and is seen with primary growths of stomach, breast, prostate and pancreas as well. It is usually thought to be due to bloodborne emboli to the lung, because in many cases tumour cells can be found in the pulmonary arteries, having reached them via the thoracic duct and systemic veins. At other times, particularly in unilateral cases, it is due to diffuse retrograde lymphatic permeation associated with obstruction to lymph flow.

Invasion of the pulmonary veins is very common and this leads to dissemination via the systemic arteries. Bloodstream spread occurs in all histological types, but is most common in oat cell tumours. The organs most frequently involved by metastases are liver, adrenals, brain, bones and kidneys.

Clinical Features

The symptoms of bronchial carcinoma arise in three main ways:

1. From the local disease—the primary tumour and adjacent lymph nodes.

2. From metastases.

3. From non-metastatic extrathoracic syndromes.

Local Disease

It may present as:

1. A finding on a routine radiograph.

2. Cough or worsening of existing cough.

3. Haemoptysis.

4. Breathlessness. This can result from collapse of a lobe or of the lung, from a pleural effusion or from replacement and compression of the lung by very large growths. Dyspnoea may also be due to a pericardial effusion or to atrial fibrillation secondary to malignant infiltration of the pericardium. Lymphangitis carcinomatosa usually causes severe breathlessness, and symptoms may be prominent even before there is much abnormality on the radiograph. Compression of the trachea will cause stridor and dyspnoea.

5. Chest pain. This may result from involvement of the pleura or from lobar collapse, both of which will cause pain on breathing, and sometimes a vague deep-seated ache in the region of the tumour is described by the patient. Involvement of intercostal nerves will give pain around the side of the chest.

6. Arm pain. Involvement of the brachial plexus by tumours at the apex of the lung can give pain in the arm and shoulder (Pancoast tumours).

7. Superior vena caval obstruction (Plate 10). Tumours and involved lymph nodes above the right hilum can obstruct the vena cava, and the patient may present with facial swelling which is particularly prominent in the mornings and relieved initially by standing. A sensation of fullness in the head is a common symptom that is described and in florid cases there will be chemosis, cyanosis and swelling of the arms and hands, with distension of the neck veins and those of the upper chest.

8. Hoarseness of the voice. Tumour at the left hilum can interrupt the recurrent laryngeal nerve and cause a vocal cord palsy. This is easily recognizable by indirect laryngoscopy.

9. Dysphagia. Involvement of the oesophagus by lymph nodes is a common event, but this symptom can also result from neurological disease such as bulbar palsy.

10. Horner's syndrome. Involvement of the inferior cervical sympathetic ganglion results in ptosis, a small pupil and anhydrosis on the same side.

Metastases

Almost any symptom may result but the following are some of the common ones:

1. Bone pain and pathological fractures.

2. Spinal cord compression leading to limb weakness.

3. Intracranial secondaries, leading to neurological deficit such as cranial nerve palsies and progressive hemiplegia. Frontal lobe tumours may produce personality change and confusion.

Headache from raised intracranial pressure can be caused by large expanding tumours or from an internal hydrocephalus from obstruction to the flow of cerebrospinal fluid.

4. Jaundice from liver metastases or obstruction of the bile duct by lymph nodes.

5. Skin secondaries, felt as nodules of variable size and appearance and often multiple.

Non-metastatic Extrapulmonary Manifestations (the Paramalignant Syndromes)

These are the disorders which are not due to the mechanical effect of either the primary tumour or its metastases, but in which the mechanism is often not known.

The incidence of these syndromes varies considerably amongst published series and appears to vary with the stage of the disease, the histology and with the degree of investigation that is undertaken.

The Endocrine Manifestations

Hypercalcaemia. This is associated with squamous cell carcinoma. The incidence is probably in the order of five to ten per cent and appears to be greatest in patients with more advanced disease. However, it is very difficult in this group to be sure that bony metastases are not present.

There are often no symptoms, but if the calcium is sufficiently high there can be confusion and drowsiness, thirst, polyuria and vomiting.

Removal of the tumour and radiotherapy cause the serum calcium to fall promptly. Corticosteroids in high doses (e.g. 60 mg prednisolone daily) are effective in approximately half of the patients.

The other endocrine manifestations usually occur with anaplastic, particularly oat cell, tumours.

Ectopic ACTH production. It is unusual to develop clinical Cushing's syndrome, probably because the patient does not live long enough to develop the features. The hypokalaemia may be profound enough to result in muscle weakness and skin pigmentation may occur, but the syndrome is usually a biochemical one and is identified by the hypokalaemic alkalosis and by a raised cortisol which is not suppressed by dexamethasone.

Specific treatment is disappointing and because of the poor prognosis will often not be indicated, though the symptoms may regress after removal of the primary tumour.

Inappropriate ADH production. The hyponatraemia can cause weakness, confusion and drowsiness, and a degree of illness that is out of proportion to the apparent extent of the disease. Water restriction and fludrocortisone have been advocated, but these do not usually lead to symptomatic improvement and oral or intravenous sodium is ineffective. Both radiotherapy and resection can be effective in abolishing the hyponatraemia. Recent studies have shown promising results with Demeclocycline 600–1200 mg daily.

Carcinoid syndrome. This is recorded in oat cell carcinomas and some carcinoid adenomas.

Gynaecomastia. This can occur in isolation or in association with hypertrophic pulmonary osteoarthropathy.

Hyperthyroidism. This is due to TSH secretion. The eye signs of thyrotoxicosis do not generally occur.

Hypoglycaemia. This is a rare manifestation of bronchial carcinoma.

Calcitonin secretion. Seventy-five per cent of oat cell carcinomas and over 40 per cent of squamous carcinomas produce the peptide hormone calcitonin. This is not associated with hypocalcaemia or other clinical findings, but plasma calcitonin assays may prove useful in following the response to treatment.

The Neurological Syndromes

Over 50 per cent of carcinomatous neuromyopathies are due to bronchial carcinoma and these occur particularly with the oat cell type. They may precede other evidence of lung cancer by several years.

1. Peripheral neuropathy (usually of mixed motor and sensory type).

2. Cerebellar degeneration.

3. Dementia.

4. A myelopathy resembling motor neurone disease.

5. Proximal myopathy. This may be difficult to distinguish from the wasting of malignant disease, but is often associated with a neuropathy.

6. Myasthenia. This is often associated with a myopathy (Eaton–Lambert syndrome), and the wasting and loss of reflexes, together with the poor response to anticholinesterase drugs, help to differentiate it from myasthenia gravis. Recognition of this syndrome is of more than academic importance because the abnormal sensitivity to muscle relaxants leads to complications during anaesthesia.

7. Polymyositis and dermatomyositis.

The Skin Manifestations

1. Dermatomyositis. Lung cancer is one of the commonest associated malignancies.

2. Acanthosis nigricans. This is usually a sign of intra-abdominal adenocarcinoma, but can be a manifestation of lung cancer.

3. Intra-epidermal skin carcinoma (Bowen's disease). A large proportion of patients with this condition develop another malignancy, including lung cancer.

Vascular Manifestations

1. Thrombophlebitis migrans is associated with mucus-secreting adenocarcinomas which are usually gastrointestinal, but can be of bronchial origin.

2. Non-bacterial thrombotic endocarditis may be secondary to bronchial carcinoma.

Hypertrophic Pulmonary Osteoarthropathy (HPOA)

HPOA is the syndrome of finger clubbing, periostitis and arthropathy. It can be caused by any of the conditions causing finger clubbing, but it is most often due to squamous cell or adenocarcinoma of the bronchus.

Together with obvious finger clubbing there is joint pain and swelling, often in the knee or ankle, and radiographs show subperiostial new bone formation at the ends of the long bones in the affected area. Gynaecomastia is present in about eight per cent of cases. The cause of the syndrome has still not been elucidated although there is evidence of both a humoral and a neural mechanism.

Nephrotic Syndrome

A membranous glomerulonephritis can occur and is often thought to result from the deposition of tumour antigen–antibody complexes on the glomerular basement membrane.

Diagnosis

The diagnosis of bronchial carcinoma can never be certain without histological or cytological confirmation, and it is an advantage to know the cell type since the prognosis will vary accordingly and the treatment will differ to some extent.

This confirmation is not, however, always necessary. In some patients it may be little more than academic because of the degree of illness or because no therapeutic implications will result. In other patients the clinical and radiological features may be sufficiently suggestive for appropriate therapy to be initiated without histology.

Sputum Cytology

It is essential that fresh, and preferably early morning, specimens of sputum are examined, and expert cytologists can then confirm the diagnosis in over 50 per cent of cases (Plate 11). Three specimens should be sent for investigation and the cytologist should be informed of any other disease which might affect interpretation, for example TB, bronchiectasis, or pulmonary fibrosis. It is important that specimens are obtained prior to bronchoscopy.

Bronchoscopy

Bronchoscopy often enables the lesion to be biopsied directly and since most tumours are relatively proximal the yield of positive biopsies is high—in the order of 60 to 70 per cent. The fibreoptic bronchoscope is better for the more peripheral lesions and for upper lobe lesions, but the size of the biopsy specimen is much smaller.

Material aspirated from the bronchial tree or obtained by a brush can be used for cytology.

Apart from obtaining histological material, bronchoscopy will show the presence of vocal cord paralysis, rigidity of the bronchus and evidence of compression by lymph nodes, and therefore give guidance as to the resectability of a lesion and also of the imminence of tracheal or main bronchial stenosis (Plates 12 and 13).

Transbronchial biopsy, which is a technique where the biopsy forceps are advanced through the bronchial wall, is being used mainly for diffuse lung lesions, but may be useful in the diagnosis of bronchial carcinoma.

Needle Biopsy

A number of different needles are available for biopsy but they are either aspiration needles, giving material for cytology, or biopsy needles which give specimens which are suitable for histology. These methods are most suitable for lesions which are too peripheral to be reached by the bronchoscope. The main complication is pneumothorax (in about 20 per cent of cases), but brisk haemorrhage can also occur.

Pleural Biopsy

The presence of a pleural effusion often means that the pleura has been invaded, and sometimes this can be demonstrated by finding malignant cells in the pleural fluid. Aspiration of the fluid can be combined with biopsy of the parietal pleura using an Abram's needle and a positive biopsy obtained in up to 60 per cent of cases.

Thoracoscopy and direct biopsy are more reliable, but are more invasive procedures.

Mediastinoscopy

The instrument is introduced through an incision in the suprasternal notch and passed downwards through the fascial planes. Biopsies are taken from mediastinal lymph nodes. Some surgeons advocate the routine use of this procedure before considering thoracotomy because of its use in assessing operability.

Other Methods

Histological material can be obtained from involved supraclavicular lymph nodes, skin metastases, bone marrow and from other involved tissues.

Treatment

The three types of specific treatment for bronchial carcinoma are surgery, radiotherapy and chemotherapy. In many patients it may not be appropriate to give any of these treatments, either because the patient is asymptomatic and unsuitable for surgery or because in the symptomatic patient other measures may be more suitable for the relief of symptoms.

Surgery

Removal of the tumour gives the best chance of a cure but in only one-quarter of the patients is a satisfactory resection possible, either because of unsuitability of the patient due to age, breathlessness or poor general health, or because of the presence of metastases or extensive local spread of the lesion. Extensive mediastinal lymph node involvement, involvement of the recurrent laryngeal and phrenic nerves and superior vena caval obstruction are all indications that satisfactory removal of the lesion is not possible, but localized involvement of the chest wall is not necessarily a contraindication to surgery. Pleural effusions are not always a result of malignant infiltration and if the effusion is clear and no malignant cells are found in the fluid or on biopsy, the lesion may still be resectable. If the fluid does not recur after aspiration this suggests that the effusion was innocent, but a recurrent effusion is almost always malignant.

Radiotherapy

Radical radiotherapy gives a better survival rate than surgery for operable oat cell carcinomas, but the results are still extremely poor, with only 10 per cent of patients surviving for two years. The results for operable squamous carcinomas are far inferior to those of surgery.

The mortality of patients with inoperable cancer is little improved by radiotherapy, so that in this group it is important that the aim of treatment should be clearly defined before it is started, and referral for radiotherapy should not be made simply because a tumour is irresectable.

Certain symptoms can be relieved or prevented by radiotherapy and regression of superficial lymph nodes and tumour masses can be achieved. Superior vena caval obstruction is best managed with radiotherapy and it is useful in relieving compression of the oesophagus, trachea or main bronchi, in reducing troublesome cough and haemoptysis and in helping bone pain. It is worth trying in some of the paramalignant syndromes if the symptoms are distressing. None of these developments is an absolute indication for radiotherapy, however, and since the treatment can cause discomfort and may involve daily travel, alternative symptomatic treatment, such as analgesics, may be more appropriate at times.

There is sometimes a place for radiotherapy after resection of a lesion if this has been incomplete, or if at thoracotomy there are indications that obstruction of such organs as bronchi or vena cava is imminent.

Chemotherapy

Chemotherapy is sometimes successful in relieving certain symptoms and in causing temporary reduction of tumour size. The small cell carcinoma responds better than the other histological types, and a variety of agents and combinations have been used. None of the drug regimens has been shown to be clearly superior to the others and there is no way of predicting whether the patient's tumour will respond. In view of the toxicity of these agents and the unreliability of their effects, most physicians reserve chemotherapy for patients who are symptomatic, whose symptoms are unsuitable for treatment by radiotherapy, but in whom there is nevertheless a reasonable life expectancy.

11. Other Malignant Tumours

Alveolar Cell Carcinoma

Alveolar cell carcinoma accounts for less than one per cent of lung cancers. It is of interest that a histologically similar condition occurring in sheep and some other animals appears to be an infectious disease. There is no evidence that human alveolar cell carcinoma is transmissible.

The cause of alveolar cell carcinoma is not known, but there is a tendency for it to occur in patients with interstitial fibrosis of any cause. The tumour appears to arise from the alveolar cells, and histologically it can be difficult to distinguish from primary or secondary adenocarcinoma.

While the tumour is small there may be no symptoms, and it is unfortunate that the diagnosis is usually delayed until the disease is widespread and is causing coughing and breathlessness. There is often production of mucoid sputum, but although a copious bronchorrhoea has been described in this condition, it is more likely to be a result of pulmonary metastases from a mucus-secreting adenocarcinoma. Radiologically it appears initially as a single nodule, but by the time symptoms have developed there is usually a diffuse nodular or pneumonia-like infiltration, often affecting both lungs. The appearances may at first suggest pulmonary metastases but tuberculosis and sarcoidosis may be involved in the differential diagnosis.

Surgical excision of the early lesion is the only effective treatment but if this is not possible, symptomatic treatment alone can be given, because the tumour does not respond to radiotherapy or chemotherapy. A temporary response to steroids is occasionally seen and a trial is worthwhile.

Mesothelioma

This malignant tumour arises from the pleura and 90 per cent are related to asbestos exposure. A previous history of occupational exposure to asbestos is often obtained, but this need not necessarily be heavy or prolonged and there can be a delay of up to 40 years from the initial exposure to the mesothelioma. The tumour usually presents with chest pain or with a pleural effusion. The diagnosis can be confirmed by needle biopsy or by open biopsy. Some tumours contain a large amount of fibrous tissue and histological diagnosis may be difficult (Plate 14). The tumour is locally invasive, and rarely metastasizes. It is common for it to infiltrate around the pleura and along the fissures, and it can invade the lung. It often spreads downwards through the diaphragm to involve the liver.

The radiological appearances are either of an irregular pleural shadow or of a pleural effusion. The early lesion resembles the benign pleural plaque, but the malignant nature will become apparent on serial radiographs.

Mesotheliomas are hardly ever amenable to resection and attempts to remove them and even diagnostic biopsies appear to worsen the already poor prognosis. Chemotherapy and radiotherapy are ineffective in arresting progression and in relieving symptoms. The pain resulting from invasion of local structures is often difficult to control and responds poorly to radiotherapy. If it is apparent that the patient is likely to survive more than a month or two, then referral to a neurosurgeon for cordotomy is often the most effective means of controlling the pain. Pleural effusions can of course be aspirated if breathlessness is a problem.

A similar tumour occurs in the peritoneum as a result of asbestos exposure and the patient presents with abdominal swelling due to ascites or with pain.

Pulmonary Lymphomas

Hodgkin's disease, the non-Hodgkin's lymphomas and chronic lymphatic leukaemia commonly involve the mediastinum. The mediastinal lymph node enlargement can be quite symptomless, but it may cause obstruction of the bronchi leading to lobar consolidation and collapse. The thoracic duct can be involved and the consequent leakage of lymph results in a milky pleural effusion—chylothorax.

Involvement of the lung itself by lymphomas can take the form of localized shadows, which sometimes cavitate, or diffuse lesions which give the appearance of consolidation. It is often difficult to know if these parenchymal shadows are due to opportunist infection or to the disease itself, but the latter is usually the case. Lung biopsy may be necessary to exclude tuberculosis and other inflammatory disorders. Similarly, when pleural effusion develops it is not easy to determine the cause.

A lateral radiograph may show the lymph node shadowing to be extending anteriorly into the retrosternal space, and this feature is useful in distinguishing the lymphomas from sarcoidosis.

Pulmonary Metastases

The lung is one of the commonest sites for metastases and a chest radiograph should be taken in all patients who are suspected of having malignant disease.

Tumours of the following origins are those most usually encountered: breast, bowel, bone, thyroid, kidney, prostate, ovary and testis.

Metastases may be demonstrated on the radiograph without there being respiratory symptoms, but the patient can develop most of the symptoms described with the local lesion of bronchial carcinoma, with cough, haemoptysis and breathlessness being the most frequent.

The radiographic appearances can be very diverse. Multiple rounded shadows are the easiest to recognize as metastases, but hydatid cysts, multiple hamartomas and rheumatoid nodules may need to be considered. The shadows are usually of varying size, reflecting the different stages of growth, but sometimes there may be a mass of small nodules of similar size, and it may be difficult to exclude miliary tuberculosis, sarcoidosis, a diffuse lobular pneumonia or even pulmonary oedema. The appearance can also resemble that of alveolar cell carcinoma. The single rounded metastasis cannot easily be distinguished from a second primary tumour. Finger clubbing can occur with both.

None of the radiological features is diagnostic of a particular tissue of origin, but the rounded 'cannon-ball' secondaries suggest kidney, bone or testis. Calcification occurs mostly with osteogenic sarcoma, and the diffuse nodular pattern usually turns out to be from the large bowel or thyroid. Pleural effusions arise mainly from the breast.

It is useful to identify prostate and kidney metastases because hormonal treatment can benefit the patient, so that it is reasonable to measure the acid phosphatase and to do a pyelogram. Apart from these there are not likely to be any therapeutic implications in identifying the primary site and exhaustive attempts to do so should be resisted.

The solitary secondary is often amenable to resection, but before it is removed, both lungs should be examined by tomography in an attempt to exclude other metastases, and thus avoid unnecessary surgery.

Tumours Which can be Malignant

Thymoma

Tumours of the thymus can be benign or malignant, but it is often difficult to determine whether a tumour is malignant, even when histology is available. The tumour can present as a finding on a radiograph, or because of compression of trachea or oesophagus, and sometimes of vena cava. It may also be found during the investigation of associated diseases such as myasthenia gravis, hypogammaglobulinaemia and red cell aplasia.

On the radiograph the tumour shows as a shadow in the upper mediastinum, and may appear to be unilateral. The lateral view shows it to be anterior. Calcification can occur.

Treatment should be surgical if possible, because there can never be certainty of the tumour being benign.

Bronchial Adenoma

These are not common and in the average thoracic surgical unit there is one for every 20 carcinomas. Most of them (90 per cent) are carcinoid tumours, although it is very rare for them to give rise to the carcinoid syndrome. The remainder are cylindromata. Although they are usually benign, both tumours can become malignant and the cylindroma is particularly prone to be locally invasive. Both types can metastasize.

They usually present with cough, haemoptysis or with pneumonia due to partial obstruction of a bronchus. Tumours of the trachea or main bronchus may cause a wheeze which is thought initially to be due to asthma. The tumour itself is often not visible on the radiograph and is diagnosed at bronchoscopy where it appears as an intraluminal tumour which can be very vascular (Plate 15).

Teratodermoid Tumours

These tumours arise from the three germinal layers and are situated in the anterior mediastinum. They can be solid tumours (teratomata) in which case malignant change is likely, or cystic (dermoids) when only about one-third become malignant. This malignant transformation is virtually restricted to males.

Because of the origin of these tumours, differentiation into almost any tissue can occur in the tumour, and this is more obvious in the cystic variety. It is not uncommon to find areas of skin, bone, hair, teeth, glandular epithelium and nerve tissue.

They present as a radiographic finding of a well-defined anterior mediastinal shadow often with calcification, or as a result of infection of the tumour or with symptoms from invasion of local structures due to malignant change. The tumour should be removed if possible.

12. Mainly Benign Tumours

Neurogenic Tumours

Neurogenic tumours arise from intercostal nerves (neurilemmoma and neurofibroma) or from a sympathetic ganglion (ganglioneuroma) and are situated posteriorly and in the paravertebral region. Symptoms may arise from pressure on the spinal cord when part of the tumour extends into an intervertebral foramen (the dumb-bell tumour), but often these tumours can be an enormous size without producing symptoms. They are usually single, but there may be more than one when there is neurofibromatosis (Von Recklinghausen's disease).

If a tumour is quite symptomless, some physicians would favour radiological review at intervals, and removal in the event of rapid increase in size or pressure symptoms. There is, however, a view that they should all be removed because the diagnosis can never be certain and because the neurofibroma can undergo sarcomatous change.

Hamartoma

A hamartoma is a benign tumour of the lung, usually containing a lot of cartilage (Plate 16). It is usually symptomless and is detected on routine radiography. It appears as a well circumscribed, rounded shadow, and often contains flecks of calcification. The usual size is one to two cm at the time of recognition and the tumour tends to enlarge slowly. There may be multiple tumours.

The differential diagnosis is usually between tuberculoma, and primary and secondary carcinoma, although the appearance may resemble that of a hydatid cyst or arteriovenous malformation.

Diagnosis is usually confirmed after removal of the lesion. There is really no alternative to surgery because it is never possible to exclude primary carcinoma, even if the lesion is calcified.

Angioma (Arteriovenous Fistula)

Angioma is in fact a malformation and not a tumour, although it appears radiographically as a rounded or lobulated shadow. The lesions can be multiple and may be associated with congenital hereditary telangiectasia (Osler–Weber–Rendu syndrome). If a significant right to left shunt occurs, then cyanosis, polycythaemia and finger clubbing can occur, and a bruit can often be heard in the lungs if the patient holds his breath in inspiration.

If possible these malformations should be removed, because the prognosis is poor if a large shunt develops, but there may be too many of them for this to be feasible.

Acknowledgements

It is a pleasure to thank Dr A. T. M. Roberts, Dr G. Laszlo and Dr Joy Harrison for their helpful comments. I am pleased also to thank Dr R. J. Sandry and the staff of the Pathology Department, Frenchay Hospital, Bristol and Dr D. Johnson and the Cytology Laboratory, Southmead Hospital, Bristol, for their help with the illustrations. Other slides have been prepared by the Department of Medical Illustration, Frenchay Hospital, and I am grateful to Mr K. Jeyasingham for providing the pictures of the operation specimens, and to Mrs Julia Flenley for typing the manuscript.

References

Chapter 9

British Medical Council, BCG and vole bacillus vaccines in the prevention of tuberculosis in adolescence and early adult life, *Br. Med. J.*, 1963, 1, 973.

East African/British Medical Research Council, Fifth investigation—third report, *Tubercle*, 1973, **54**, 169.

Frimodt-Møller, J., Thomas, J., and Parthasarathy, R., Observation on the protective effect of BCG vaccination in a South Indian rural population, Bull. Wld. Hlth. Org., 1964, **30**, 545.

Rosenthal, S. R., Loewinsohn, E., Graham, M. L., Liveright, D., Thorne, M. C., Johnson, V., and Batson, H. C., BCG vaccination against tuberculosis in Chicago. A 20 year study statistically analysed, *Paediatrics*, 1961, **28**, 622.

Chapter 10

Bryson, C. C. and Spencer, H., *Quart. Med. J.*, 1951, **20** NS, 173.

Caplin, M. Tumours of the Lung, *Medicine*, 1972, **14**, 919.

Doll, R. and Hill, A. B., A study of the aetiology of carcinoma of the lung, *Br. Med. J.*, 1952, **2**, 1271.

Nicholson, W. F., Fox, M. and Bryce, A. G., Review of 910 cases of bronchial carcinoma with results of treatment, *Lancet*, 1957, **i**, 296.

Further Reading

Crofton, J. and Douglas, A., *Respiratory Diseases*, 2nd ed., Blackwell, Oxford, 1975.

Garrod, L. P., Lambert, H. P. and O'Grady, F., *Antibiotic Chemotherapy*, 4th ed., Churchill Livingstone, London and Edinburgh, 1973.

Parkes, W. R., *Occupational Lung Disorders*, Butterworth, London, 1975.

Spencer, H., *Pathology of the Lung*, 3rd ed., Pergamon Press, Oxford, 1977.

Index